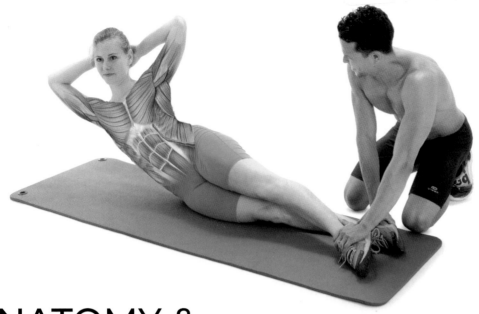

ANATOMY &
STRENGTH TRAINING
WITHOUT SPECIALIZED
EQUIPMENT

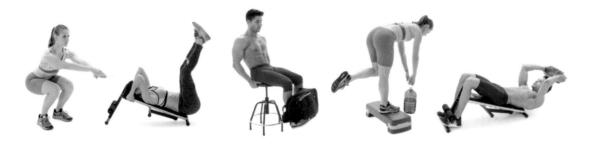

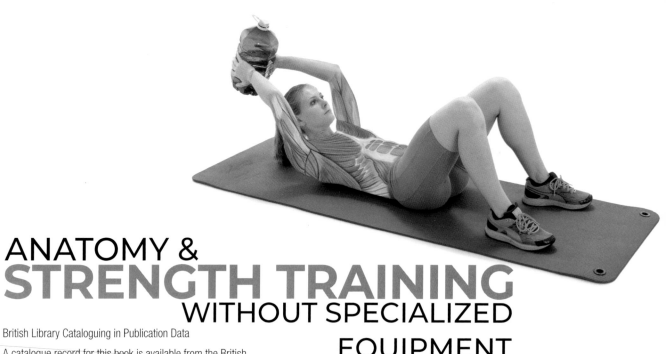

ANATOMY &
STRENGTH TRAINING
WITHOUT SPECIALIZED
EQUIPMENT

British Library Cataloguing in Publication Data

A catalogue record for this book is available from the British Library

Anatomy & Strength Training

Maidenhead: Meyer & Meyer Sport (UK) Ltd., 2020

ISBN: 978-1-78255-193-5

Aachen, Auckland, Beirut, Cairo, Cape Town, Dubai, Hägendorf, Hong Kong, Indianapolis, Manila, New Delhi, Singapore, Sydney, Tehran, Vienna

Member of the World Sports Publishers' Association (WSPA), www.w-s-p-a.org

Printed in Spain

ISBN: 978-1-78255-193-5

Email: info@m-m-sports.com
www.thesportspublisher.com

Managing editor: Elizabeth Evans

Copyeditor: Qurratulain Zaheer

Translator: AAA Translations, St. Louis, MO

Typsetting: Zerosoft

Original version:
Anatomia & Musculacion Sin Aparatos, © 2019 Editorial Paidotribo —World Rights Published by Editorial Paidotribo, Spain

Project and execution: Editorial Paidotribo

Editorial Direction: María Fernanda Canal

We would like to thank Luis Martinez (ADEP, Miguel Angel Segura (Bcn 24 h fitness) for l us their athletic facilities to shoot the photog that appear in this book. Without their object collaboration, this project would not have be to be brought to a successful end.

Text: Guillermo Seijas

Scientific Review: Victor Gôtzens

Revising: Roser Pérez

Graphic design: Toni Inglès

Illustrations: Myriam Ferron

Photos: Nos i Soto, Manuel Albir

Layout: Estudi Toni Inglès Models: Francisco Jes Lozano, Gerardo Valera, Goretti Cela, Guillermo S Mireia Asensio, Viktoria Kohalmi

Pre-printing: Estudi Genís

Production: Sagrafic, S.L.

Printed in Spain

Preface

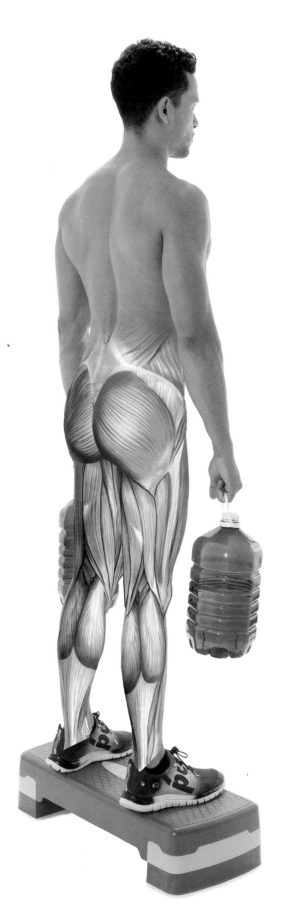

E There are many reasons why an athlete may wish to try bodybuilding without specific devices or materials.

Perhaps it is his first time bodybuilding and he believes that a good way to begin is to exercise almost alone, using only his body weight and a good exercise routine.

Perhaps he is an advanced athlete just looking for a change, or someone who feels he can't "tie himself down" to a fitness center. These are only a few examples of why an athlete may seek a new form of exercise.

What is certain is that, if he wishes to try this route, this book will be of great help to him. In these pages, we will attempt to teach or remind you of several basic concepts for bodybuilding training of which you may not be aware, or that you have left by the wayside when facing the monotony that training can become.

Sometimes, it is a good idea to pause and ask yourself if what you are doing makes sense and is helping you to improve, or if it is simply an accepted habit that you no longer think about, because it is convenient, or because you have been doing this all your life.

Whether you are seeking new exercises to make your training sessions more entertaining and variable, or you need some routines to introduce yourself to bodybuilding, or even if you need to turn your athletic habits upside down, you will find the resources to do so in this book.

You will not find stories from the gym, unfounded anonymous beliefs supported by nothing but personal hunches. In fact, it is very much the opposite. In order to present this book, we used current data, some of the latest studies regarding hypertrophic training, and the latest bodybuilding publications by specialists of recognized importance.

But you must not think that this book arose solely from data extraction and reading, since its authors also have lengthy practical experience with bodybuilding training and with training professionals in this field.

If you have the necessary motivation and perseverance, this book will give you the tools to achieve your best body.

Contents

How to use this book

EXERCISE

Exercise number

Area worked

Muscle worked

Exercise name

DESCRIPTION OF THE EXERCISE

Description of the exercise

Level of difficulty

Execution of the exercise

Starting position

Technical advice

Final position

Muscles worked in color

Muscles worked in bold type

Other muscles distinguished in the area worked

MUSCLES WORKED

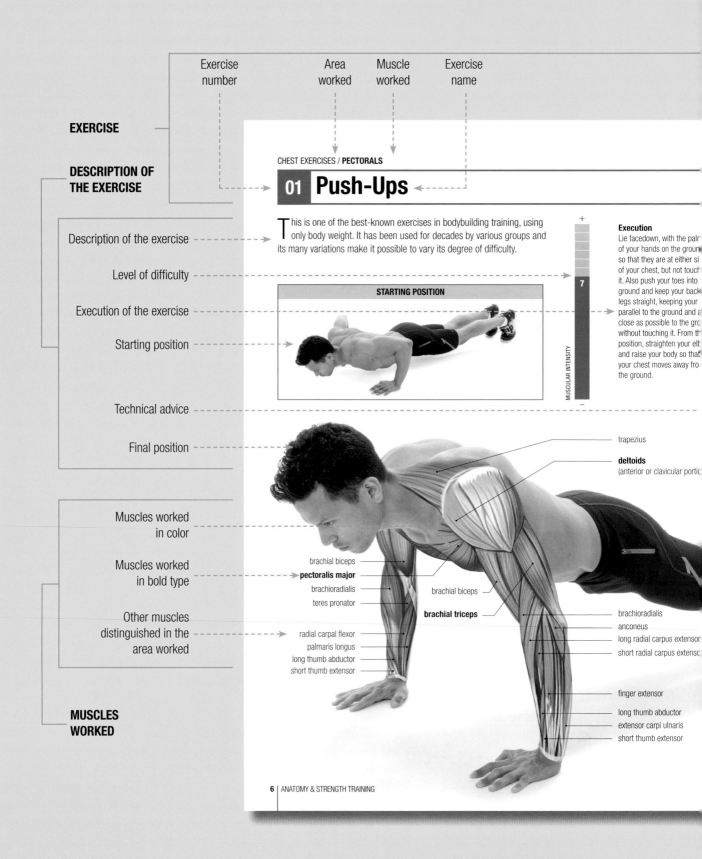

CHEST EXERCISES / **PECTORALS**

01 Push-Ups

This is one of the best-known exercises in bodybuilding training, using only body weight. It has been used for decades by various groups and its many variations make it possible to vary its degree of difficulty.

STARTING POSITION

MUSCULAR INTENSITY

7

Execution
Lie facedown, with the palm of your hands on the groun so that they are at either si of your chest, but not touch it. Also push your toes into ground and keep your back legs straight, keeping your parallel to the ground and a close as possible to the gro without touching it. From th position, straighten your elk and raise your body so that your chest moves away fro the ground.

trapezius

deltoids
(anterior or clavicular portic

brachial biceps

pectoralis major

brachioradialis

teres pronator

brachial biceps

brachial triceps

brachioradialis
anconeus
long radial carpus extensor
short radial carpus extenso

radial carpal flexor
palmaris longus
long thumb abductor
short thumb extensor

finger extensor

long thumb abductor
extensor carpi ulnaris
short thumb extensor

6 | ANATOMY & STRENGTH TRAINING

Easier and
harder variations

Diagram of the
area worked

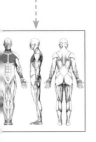

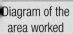

Your trunk and lower
extremities must be in
perfect alignment.

Limit the movement of your
elbows and shoulders.

Lower yourself as far as
possible without using the
ground to support your
weight.

Push Ups

ALTERNATIVE EXERCISES `01`

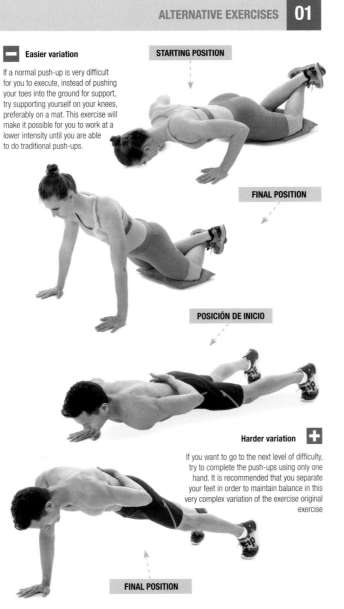

Easier variation

If a normal push-up is very difficult
for you to execute, instead of pushing
your toes into the ground for support,
try supporting yourself on your knees,
preferably on a mat. This exercise will
make it possible for you to work at a
lower intensity until you are able
to do traditional push-ups.

STARTING POSITION

FINAL POSITION

POSICIÓN DE INICIO

Harder variation +

If you want to go to the next level of difficulty,
try to complete the push-ups using only one
hand. It is recommended that you separate
your feet in order to maintain balance in this
very complex variation of the exercise original
exercise

FINAL POSITION

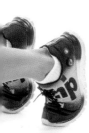

Easier
variation

Harder
variation

**TRAINING
ROUTINES**
(pages 146-151)

page

number   position

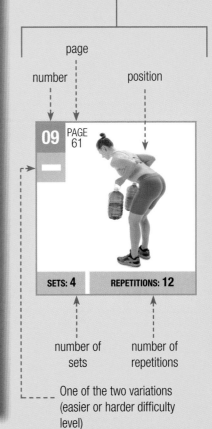

`09` PAGE
61

SETS: 4   REPETITIONS: 12

number of   number of
sets   repetitions

One of the two variations
(easier or harder difficulty
level)

The muscles

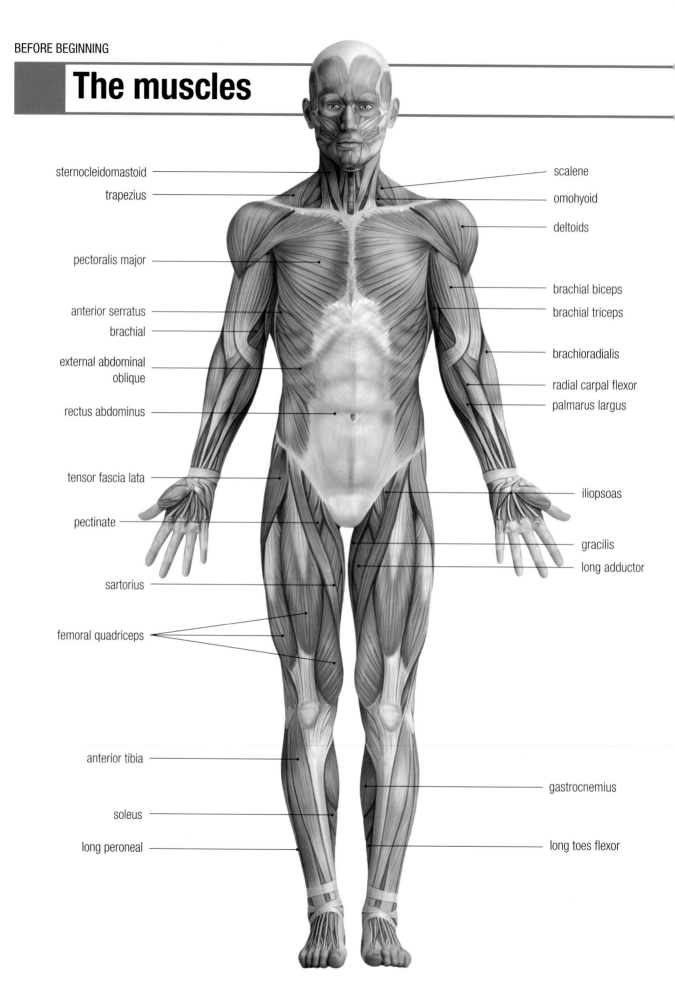

sternocleidomastoid

trapezius

pectoralis major

anterior serratus

brachial

external abdominal
oblique

rectus abdominus

tensor fascia lata

pectinate

sartorius

femoral quadriceps

anterior tibia

soleus

long peroneal

scalene

omohyoid

deltoids

brachial biceps

brachial triceps

brachioradialis

radial carpal flexor

palmarus largus

iliopsoas

gracilis

long adductor

gastrocnemius

long toes flexor

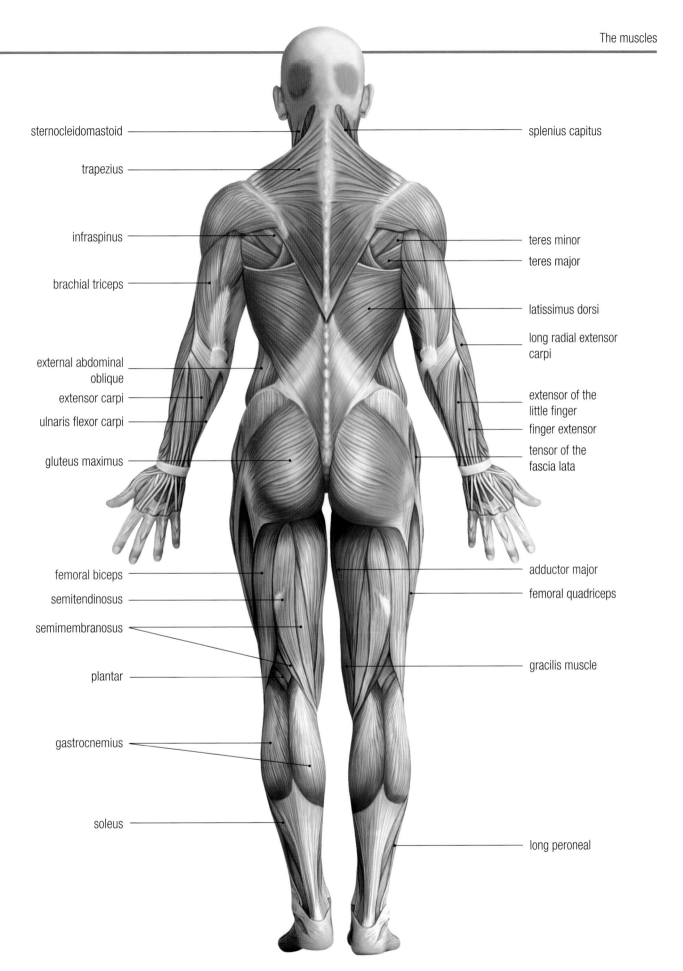

sternocleidomastoid

trapezius

infraspinus

brachial triceps

external abdominal
oblique

extensor carpi

ulnaris flexor carpi

gluteus maximus

femoral biceps

semitendinosus

semimembranosus

plantar

gastrocnemius

soleus

splenius capitus

teres minor

teres major

latissimus dorsi

long radial extensor
carpi

extensor of the
little finger

finger extensor

tensor of the
fascia lata

adductor major

femoral quadriceps

gracilis muscle

long peroneal

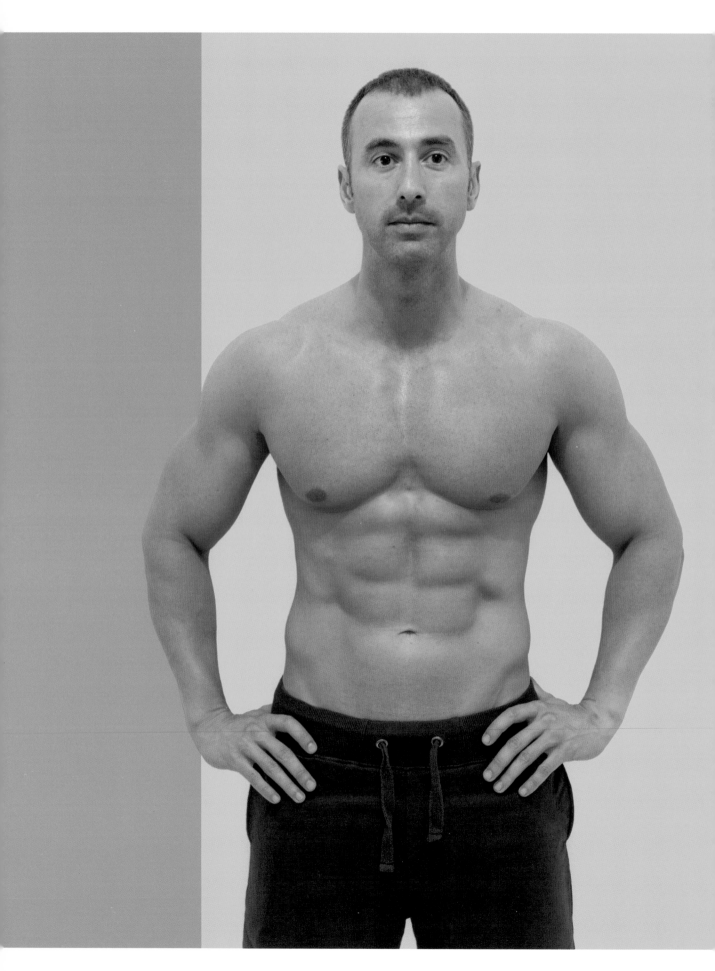

Strength training with bodyweight

Strength training is the development of skeletal muscles by the use of exercises and routines designed for this purpose. When we speak of strength training, we usually think of perfectly equipped gyms with dumbbells, benches, bars, discs, apparatuses, pulleys and a long list of specific and very expensive equipment which can only be found in fitness centers. We also think of very muscular individuals doing analytical exercises against resistance.

This traditional type of work is certainly very effective, and there is a reason for why it has been the most used for decades in order to improve muscle mass and tone.

On the other hand, there are new trends and products released every year which promise the maximum in performance, health, longevity and well-being. Some even promise results in just a few weeks, without you having to get up from the sofa, and only having to invest a few minutes a day or week. Faced with the avalanche of publicity, it is worthwhile to ask if any high performing athletes use these types of methods or products in their training sessions. Have you ever seen an elite bodybuilder develop his or her abdominals by using small electrodes that are sold on television? Probably only those who are paid to appear in the ad.

Nonetheless, it is true that many new trends have a few elements of great usefulness, and it is worthwhile to integrate these into your daily routines. Training in suspension, functional training or calisthenics, are good examples of this, especially if you have an interest in bodybuilding, but are not using it as your only goal.

In conclusion, although there is a classic method for strength training, there are also many others that provide good results, and the combination of the best of each of them will enable you to reach the goals you have set in a more varied and entertaining way.

With this book, you will learn to choose what is of benefit to you and discard the rest, only taking the different methods and trends into consideration.

What is bodyweight strength training?

Strength training has always been done with specific equipment, which is often expensive and heavy. However, in order to perform the exercises in this discipline, all you need is a resistance to overcome, which can be derived from various sources. The resistance that is within reach of everyone is one's own body weight, and various disciplines including calisthenics, are based on this element.

PUSH

The usual method of using this resistance is on the ground. Thus, with our own body weight and the ground as a point of support, it is possible to perform a multitude of pushing with resistance exercises: squats, lunges, etc.

At home, or in the city environment, there are a multitude of elements available that make it possible to vary the angle of work by introducing small changes. Thus, a wall, a bench or stairs can provide a large number of variants in the execution of a push up, making it possible to modify its difficulty or

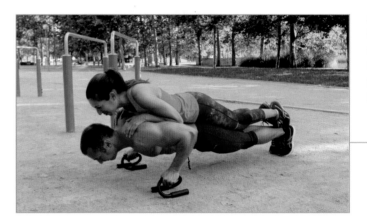

A simple exercise is a push-up which can be converted into a very difficult exercise with the help of a partner.

increase its impact on one or another area of the pectorals.

If you have the good fortune to be training with a partner, or in a group, your partner will be able to help you increase or decrease resistance.

If you cannot do this exercise alone, your partner will help you overcome the resistance by working with you, and if you find that the exercise is too easy because you are at a more advanced level, your partner can push on you or even add, part, or all of his weight to yours. In addition, training in a group is always more fun and can become a challenge because it introduces healthy competition between athletes.

There are a multitude of variants which make it possible to modify the difficulty of these exercises, for example, performing them with only one arm or leg. One-arm push ups or one-leg squats are a challenge, even for the most experienced athlete. Other variants of intermediate complexity, such as performing exercises with weighted items (a backpack full of books, a liquid container, etc.), will provide a broader range of levels of difficulty.

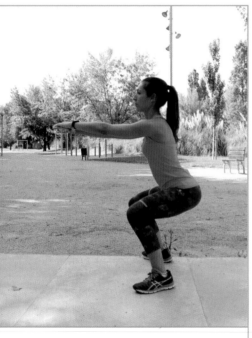

Squats are exercises that can be done with one's own body weight, although it is a good idea to add resistance as your level improves.

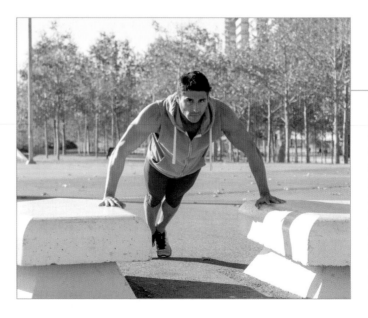

Using two benches makes it possible to work the pectorals, especially their sternocostal and abdominal portions. There is also a broader range of movement since the ground does not shorten the negative phase of the exercise.

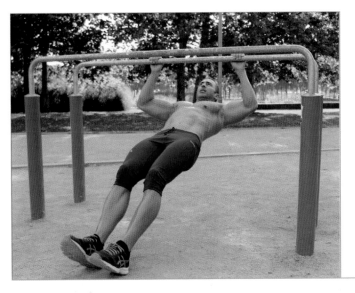

TENSION

Many muscle groups cannot be worked with pushing exercises, since their function is closely related to stretching movements; some of these muscles are the latissimus dorsi, the trapezius or the brachial biceps. One or more elements to pull will almost certainly be necessary. With very few of our own items, or with some taken from the natural or urban environment, we can make up for any lack of specialized equipment.

Many structures which can be used as bars to hang from can be found in urban and natural environments. However, before using them, it is important to define some requirements.

More and more parks and recreation areas have fixed structures for performing tension exercises. These urban elements have often been designed for this purpose.

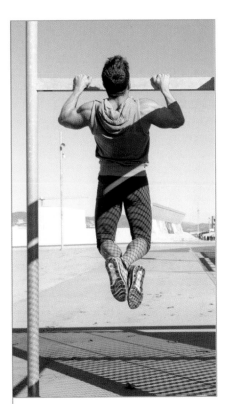

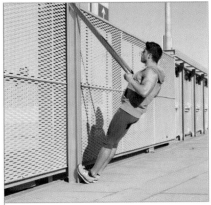

A girder and a nylon belt or cord will make it possible to do a multitude of tension exercises; one need only vary the angle of the body to increase or decrease difficulty.

• **Safety.** Any element used as a support must meet several minimum safety requirements: resistance, adequate distance from the ground, and surfaces without edges or irregularities which can damage your hands or the part of the body used as a support.

• **Suitability and durability.** Do not use elements from the environment which deteriorate due to the use we make of them, or whose use is inappropriate: it is a good idea to stay away from structures in children's parks, from traffic signals, etc.

It is a good idea to add nylon cords or belts to this suspension work. These make it possible to broaden your repertory of tension exercises to a spectacular degree, since it is enough to have a support to anchor them on in order to perform a multitude of new exercises; at times, this also makes it possible to increase your repertory of pushing exercises.

This metallic structure has appropriate resistance and durability characteristics. It is a robust support at an adequate height and does not deteriorate with use.

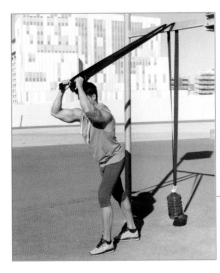

The same belt passed over a support, and with a weight at one of the ends works as a simple pulley mechanism.

Strength training with devices: pros and cons

There is no single way to increase our muscle mass. While it is true that there are ways that are more often used, or that are considered more efficient in the pursuit of this objective, there are also other paths that provide excellent results. We use the word "devices" to indicate all specialized equipment.

THE PROS OF STRENGTH TRAINING WITH DEVICES

Among the arguments that are used in favor of strength training with devices, the following stand out:

• There are a multitude of machines, benches, pulleys and other elements specifically created for bodybuilding exercises. These elements provide a broad selection of possibilities for training and meet the conditions for safety and robustness that every athlete requires.

• Working with machines guides the movement, and is a good option for beginners, or those whose technique needs work. It is almost impossible to slip out of the path marked by the machine and, in addition, the risk of harming oneself in such well-defined movements is minimal.

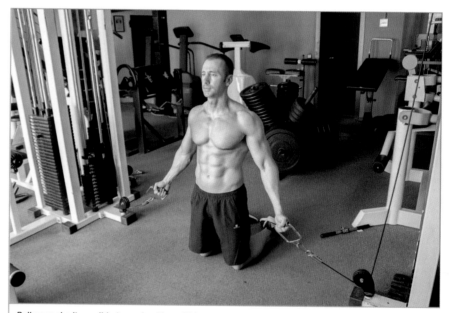

Pulleys make it possible to work with multiple angles and resistances while only moving a weight or height selector.

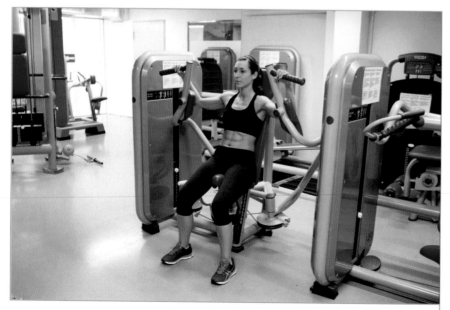

• The intensity of the work is easy to regulate, since it is sufficient to add or remove weight in each series, whether by incorporating discs, planks or even using lighter or heavier dumbbells. This makes it possible to adjust the exercise to the needs of each person, in a minimal amount of time.

• Joining a gym ensures access to a broad range of possibilities to play with and combine in order to continue adapting your routines.

• In general, the atmosphere in gyms meets the conditions for optimum temperature and ventilation, and even provides a completely equipped changing room so that comfort is clearly a point in their favor.

The majority of machines make it possible to work from a comfortable position. Their design provides a guided movement, which minimizes the effects of technical deficiencies of the athlete and the risks of injury.

THE CONS OF BODYBUILDING WITH DEVICES

Not everything about training with devices is advantageous; there are also negative aspects. These are the principal cons:

• The specialized equipment in gyms is often expensive and voluminous, making it difficult to install a complete gym in your home. The alternative is to join one, but this means paying monthly dues.

• Except for exclusive gyms, the majority of centers experience significant fluctuations in attendance, depending on the time of year and the time slot. You may be able to train easily, and pleasantly, on a morning in December but, on an afternoon in June, it may be a little less impossible; just at the moment when the efforts of your work can be best shown off, you will find significant obstacles to maintaining your exercise routine.

• If your life style involves travel, it will be impossible to get to the gym; you will have to take a break from your work routine every time you travel, or have to pay one-time fees at gyms located in the places you travel to, if you can even get into them.

• Each gym has its own equipment and distribution; the poorly equipped ones will limit the variety of exercises you can perform, and changes from one gym to the next will force you to adapt to new devices and work areas.

• While the one-time or balanced use of machines enriches your daily routine and is beneficial to its practitioners, its abuse, or the abuse of very analytical exercises, will put the brakes on other qualities which must also be developed: balance, coordination, proprioception or improvement of technique in different exercises, among others.

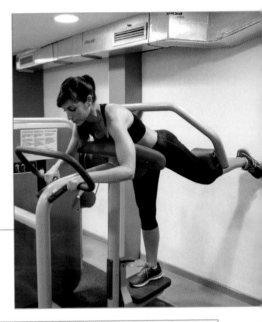

The abusive use of machines can result in a waning of technique and coordination, especially of intramuscular coordination.

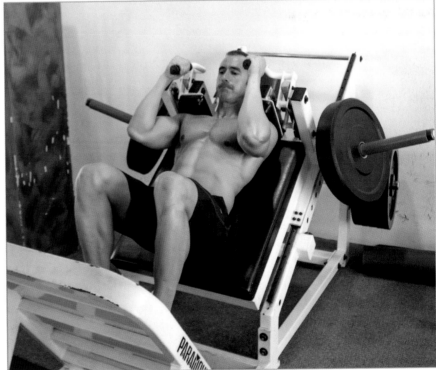

It may be that some of the options you are used to, such as this hack press, are not to be found in the majority of gyms, which can be a problem if you cannot get to your usual gym.

Strength training without devices: pros and cons

Strength training without devices has its own pros and cons. It is not our intention in this book to hide the negative aspects and put forward the positive ones, so we will try to offer an objective view of the method, without avoiding its faults. It is important to remember that the most complete training is that which takes the best from each method, and the most intelligent athlete is the one who keeps his or her mind open, without losing the critical analysis ability.

THE PROS OF STRENGTH TRAINING WITHOUT DEVICES

Principal benefits of training without devices:

• It is possible to train completely, at any time and place, with the only necessary element being your own body.
This frees you from the need to go to a center that has specific equipment.

• Anyone, including those who live in remote places or far from the services offered in large cities, can design and apply their own training routines. If, during a vacation, you decide to spend some days in a natural environment, you can continue exercising if you wish.

• It requires very little equipment which, in addition, does not need to be specific. For this reason, some elements in your home, or in an urban or natural environment, can be used for training sessions. In cases where you buy the equipment, it will be very low cost and easy to acquire or substitute for other options.

• The very broad range of existing exercises makes it possible to prepare complete training routines of lesser to greater difficulty, suited to the fitness level or experience of each practitioner. Other elements such as inclination, weights or assistance also make it possible to graduate the difficulty.

• The movements are unrestricted; this also increases strength and muscle mass, requires greater technique, coordination and body control. All of this together will help you to be a more complete and functional athlete.

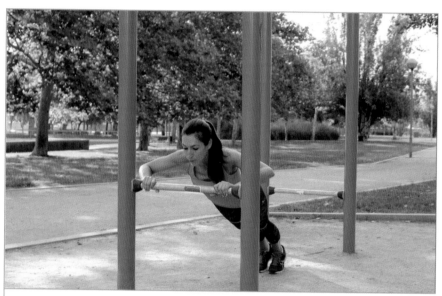

Reducing the slant of the body in a push up also lessens its difficulty.

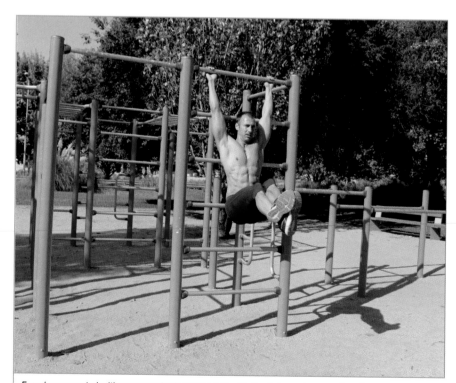

Exercises executed with your own body weight and with fixed elements, as well as those executed with free weights, improve coordination and control of your body.

THE CONS OF STRENGTH TRAINING WITHOUT DEVICES

With regard to the disadvantages of training without devices, it is appropriate to mention the weak points of this method, which, although few in number, should be kept in mind before beginning to prepare a training routine.

• In the majority of exercises performed with specific equipment, the difficulty increases from beginning levels to very advanced with the simple action of adding discs or changing one set of dumbbells for another. When doing exercises without devices, this variation can be achieved with inclination or with weights, but in 90% of cases, the ranges of difficulty are narrower and less adaptable.

• If indeed it is not necessary to go to a specific place to train, it may be that finding some of the elements to do so (fixed bars, beams, railings, benches, branches, etc.) will oblige the practitioner to travel further than she wishes.

• The practice of always training with body weight or with free weights, promotes coordination and improves the general abilities of any person; nonetheless, it can be a limiting factor for beginners, whose experience is limited, or for those who have difficulties in focusing on strength in a determined muscle group.

• Traditional equipment makes it possible to record the weights you are working with and to execute a methodical tracking of your progression, but this task is somewhat difficult when there is no specific equipment, and it is necessary to guide yourself using only your own sensations.

• The freedom with which you execute body weight movements or free weights movements can make you more vulnerable to injuries in the case of an accident or of poor execution of technique.

• Routines for the leg muscles can be limited or deficient, since it can be complicated to find resistances that make it possible to work powerful muscle groups, such as the quadriceps, at high intensity.

Training without devices, at times, cannot cover the multiple degrees of difficulty which is covered by traditional training by adding or removing weight (adding discs, planks or changing dumbbells...).

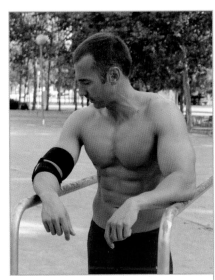

It is much easier to become injured with freedom of movement than with exercises using machines, where the movement is guided.

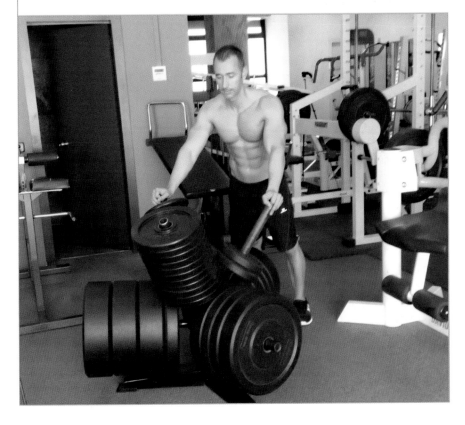

Where and how to exercise

For someone who is used to training in a gym, it may be difficult to imagine how the urban or natural environment can provide the resources you need to train in a complete and balanced way. There is no remedy for this better than a stroll through the city, which here is Barcelona and its surroundings, to discover the multitude of options which are in plain sight and often overlooked.

PARALLEL BARS

Many public parks have parallel bars for exercising, but there are also other elements in the urban environment, such as structures for parking bicycles, which can serve the same function.

BENCHES

The term "bench" not only refers to a bench, but rather to a place where it is possible to lie down to execute an exercise, for example, for abdominals.

FIXED BARS

Training without having the availability of a place from which to hang in order to do pull-ups or their variants can be difficult. Nonetheless, the urban environment is full of elements that make this task easy, while also being suited to your own possibilities and limitations, avoiding damaging the elements and complying with local regulations.

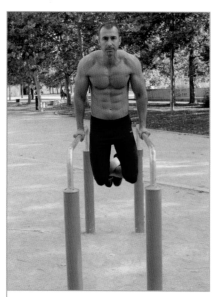

Parallel bars installed in a public park.

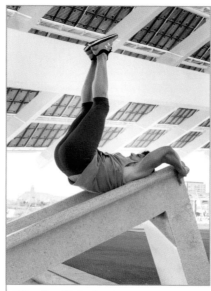

This railing fills the function of a bench and adds the element of inclination, making the exercise more difficult.

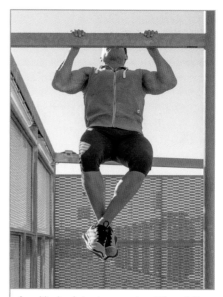

A multitude of structures such as this metallic enclosure function as fixed bars.

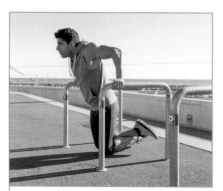

The parallel supports of a bicycle rack can be substituted for bars.

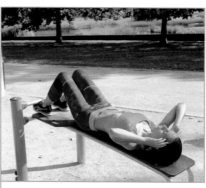

Some parks, in addition to traditional benches for sitting, provide other options which meet the same function.

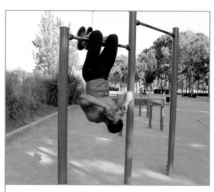

Structures with bars at different heights are more and more common in parks and beach areas.

SUPPORT POINTS OF VARYING HEIGHTS

These are a basic element for varying the difficulty of the exercises and for executing those which require that the feet be situated above the hands, or the reverse. Push-ups, triceps dips, or lunges, for example, can be executed with supports that, although not necessary, provide variety.

Two benches or seats located a short distance apart provide separated supports in the lowering portion of push-ups, and increase difficulty in triceps dips.

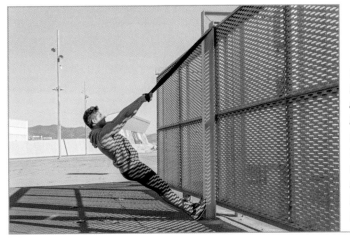

This beam fixed to the ground is used as anchoring for a belt or cord from which we can hang. This urban element does not suffer any damage from being used and is resistant.

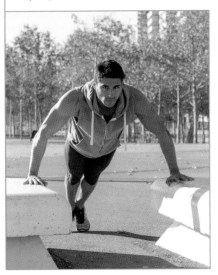

ANCHORING POINTS

Fixed points for anchoring a belt or cord, or from which to slide it, are basic elements if you want to add the multitude of exercises that suspension devices make possible to your routine. In their absence, a nylon belt or cord, which will fill the same function can be used for a much lower cost. A tree or robust branch, a beam or any other raised and resistant element will serve this purpose.

These are only a few ideas from among all of those that can be imagined. Training without devices is a form of continuous development exercise and, over long-term training sessions and the increase of your experience and improvement of your physical condition, you will modify and create your own exercises so that your training continues to be more varied and suited to your needs.

After a while, you will make modifications and adaptations to exercises naturally, and without thinking about it. You will implement new forms and discard others, embarking on a progression without limits which will turn you into an autonomous athlete and an expert on yourself.

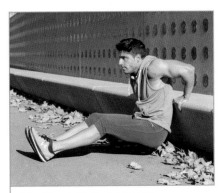

A fixed bench fills the function of a raised support.

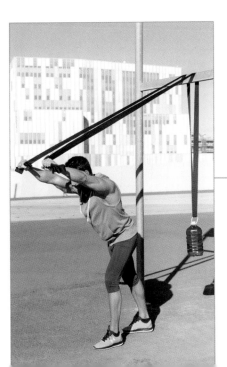

An improvised pulley can be made by hanging a weight from the opposite end of a belt and sliding it over another element.

Basic terms

Before beginning an analysis of the various principles of training and their application to training, there are several parameters to learn which are helpful in understanding later concepts, including the distribution and composition of a training routine.

TRAINING LOAD

This is the parameter that measures the stimulus to which an athlete subjects himself in order to attain a response from the body. It refers to the dimension of training stimulus and encompasses the variables that comprise it, which are **volume** and **intensity**.

Volume

This is the quantitative element; the quantity of exercise completed. In general, this quantity can be measured in kilometers, minutes, etc. For a cyclist, the volume of a training session could correspond to kilometers traveled. Bodybuilding athletes often measure in **repetitions**, **series** and **exercises**.

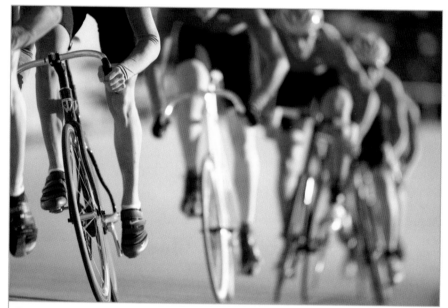

For a cyclist, the volume of training can be measured in kilometers.

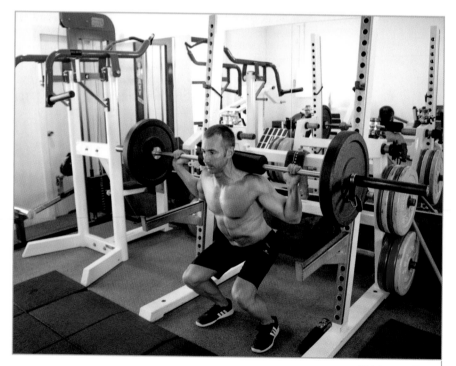

Athlete executing a repetition of a squat.

Repetition. Execution of a one bodybuilding movement. Thus, doing one squat would be to execute one repetition of the squat exercise.

Series. Group of repetitions between rests. Thus, if you execute seven squat movements and then rest, you will have executed a series of seven repetitions in the squat exercise. If you then execute seven more, you will be executing a second series. Two series of seven repetitions.

Exercise. Type of bodybuilding movement you are doing: squats, lunges, push-ups, lateral raises, etc.

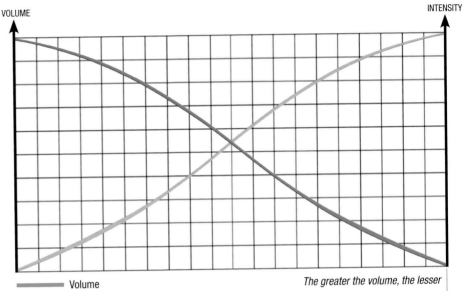

VOLUME — INTENSITY

Volume
Intensity

The greater the volume, the lesser its intensity and vice versa.

Intensity. Difficulty of the exercise is the qualitative element, which is measured in different ways. In resistance athletes, intensity is measured by heart rate. These athletes estimate their maximum heart rate as a function of their age and sex, and determine at what percentage of this maximum heart rate they wish to work. Starting from there, they use a heart rate monitor to monitor the intensity of the exercise. In bodybuilding athletes, we use a % of one maximum repetition (1RM).

1RM. This is the maximum weight that the athlete can move to complete one repetition of a determined exercise, without it being possible to do a second. Example: if you wish to work at 80% of intensity on the bench press, and you know that you lift a maximum of 100 kg in said exercise one time, you will have to work with 80 kg.

Except in the initial stages of training, it will be complicated to increase the variables of volume and intensity simultaneously. High training volumes are not compatible with high intensities and vice versa. Thus, a marathon enthusiast will be able to run for hours, which assumes a high volume, but will find it difficult to be able to maintain a velocity greater than 30 km/h.

Likewise, a sprinter will be able to run the 100 m easily at an average speed greater than 30 km/h, which assumes high intensity, but will not be able to run for 3 straight hours.

If we extrapolate to bodybuilding, it is appropriate to say that if an athlete decides to train the chest, he will be able to do so at a high intensity such as 85% of 1 RM if he wishes to complete 3 series of 10 repetitions, which is a low volume. On the other hand, if he seeks to complete 25 series of 20 repetitions each, it will be impossible to do so at an intensity of 85% of 1RM. Obviously, these examples are extreme, but they are to be considered only for clarification.

PRINCIPLES OF TRAINING

According to Müller's definition (1997), the principles of training are a "Series of hierarchically superior instructions for the activity of athletic training." Thus, they act as more of a general basis for orientation and less of a concrete guideline for the activity. That is, they are scientifically based and general standards which should be used as references when planning training sessions.

The objective of this book is bodybuilding, so we will describe the principles that we believe are most representative, without leaning exclusively on any one author, and we will relate them to their practical application in the field of bodybuilding.

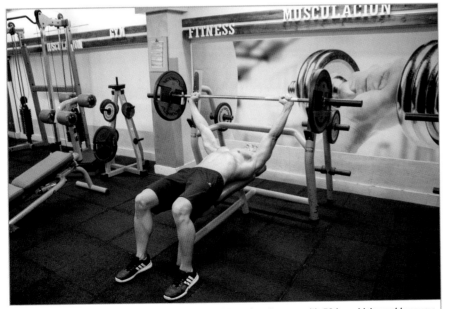

Athlete exercising a bench press with 52 kg, which would assume approximately 43% of your 1RM, and would reach 120 kg.

Principle of specificity

You will reach higher performance rates if the work you do is focused on your discipline. If you wish to achieve an ambitious objective, center each training session on improving the qualities and abilities that are of greatest importance in your exercise routine. This principle is especially applicable to those athletes who are in pursuit of excellence or at a higher athletic performance level in a specific discipline.

All athletes must establish a solid basis on which to build the first steps of their approach to physical activity. Working with different physical qualities and skills will provide you with the foundations on which to continue growing, making it possible for you to develop abilities that you will transfer to later learning.

Once you have achieved a certain level, you should concentrate on working on the qualities and abilities which will enable you to achieve the maximum level in your specialty. Including other types of work will be counterproductive if you aspire to achieve the maximum in a specific sport.

A heptathlon athlete provides a great example. She must master seven disciplines: 100 m hurdles, 200 m dash, 800 m dash, high vault, long jump, shot put and the javelin throw. An athlete who achieves high performance in all of these areas is an all-around athlete. But, if you have to compete separately in each specialty against the specialists in each one, you would probably come in in last place in every competition.

The heptathlon athlete is probably more well-rounded than the shot putter, but it would be harder for her to beat him in his own specialty.

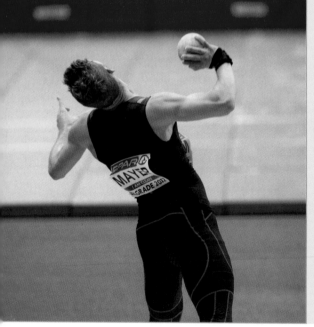

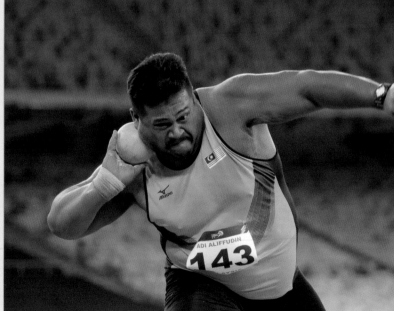

In the strength training world, there is an eternal debate regarding whether it is advisable or counterproductive to train in combined strength training work.

This means that with aerobic work, you are doing a competing type of training. It is generally accepted that introducing aerobic work into the routine of a muscle hypertrophying athlete is something negative.

This is true up to a certain point, since the majority of studies on the subject indicate that aerobic training, if done at an intensity of 80% or greater, promotes an increase in muscle mass, especially in untrained subjects. In addition, it is known that certain anabolic markers increase after doing high intensity aerobic exercises.

On the other hand, and as framed by this principal, it seems logical to think that, long term, a single muscle will not be able to adapt itself by the typology of its fibers or by its metabolism, to both aerobic work and hypertrophy. It seems appropriate to conclude, therefore, that an athlete who wishes to achieve high performance must do so in a way in which they do not experience interference between different types of training.

Practical recommendation: given the lack of data stating that aerobic exercise is counterproductive in hypertrophying muscles, and taking into account that the risks may be minimized by doing low volumes of work and at a high intensity, we do not recommend that you eliminate this type of work. You should also remember the multiple benefits that aerobic work brings to the body. A good option would be to do short sessions of aerobic work after hypertrophy work or in independent sessions of about 30 minutes.

A non-competitive strength training athlete should not exclude brief sessions of aerobic exercise in their routines as a supplement to muscle hypertrophying training.

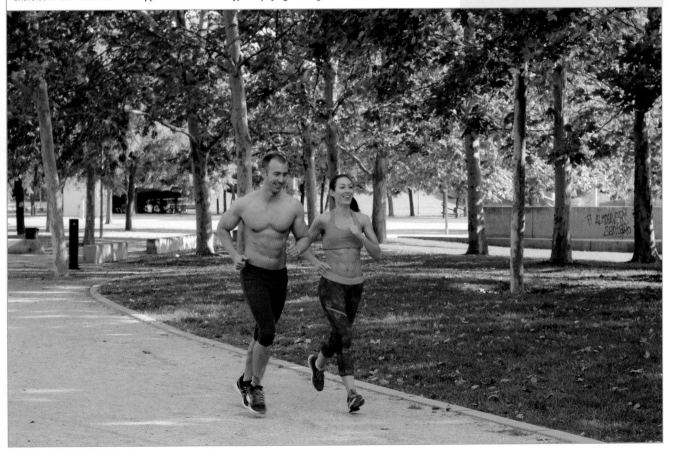

Overloading principle

Training must assume a stimulus to the body that is sufficiently great so as to generate an adaptive response, but without being so great as to cause excessive exhaustion or create conditions that make it impossible for the body to recover appropriately in a sufficient amount of time. If training is not very intense, it will not lead to improvements in the athlete, and if excessive, it will worsen their general condition. Look for the right stimulus.

The Threshold Law or Principle of Arnodt and Schultz confirms that in order for a stimulus to cause adaptations or improvements in the athlete, it must exceed a certain level or threshold, which will differ as a function of the individual characteristics of each athlete. Below this level, the stimulus will have no effect. On the other hand, all athletes have a maximum tolerance level and some stimuli exceed this excessive level of stress on the body. With this, your form deteriorates and the risk of injuries there is more of a risk of abandoning the activity.

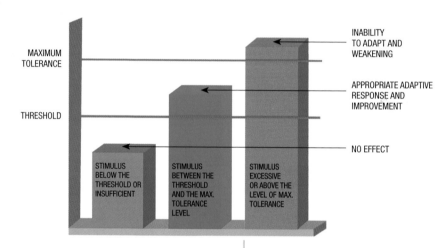

MAXIMUM TOLERANCE

THRESHOLD

INABILITY TO ADAPT AND WEAKENING

APPROPRIATE ADAPTIVE RESPONSE AND IMPROVEMENT

NO EFFECT

STIMULUS BELOW THE THRESHOLD OR INSUFFICIENT

STIMULUS BETWEEN THE THRESHOLD AND THE MAX. TOLERANCE LEVEL

STIMULUS EXCESSIVE OR ABOVE THE LEVEL OF MAX. TOLERANCE

Insufficient stimuli do not improve physical condition and excessive ones worsen it.

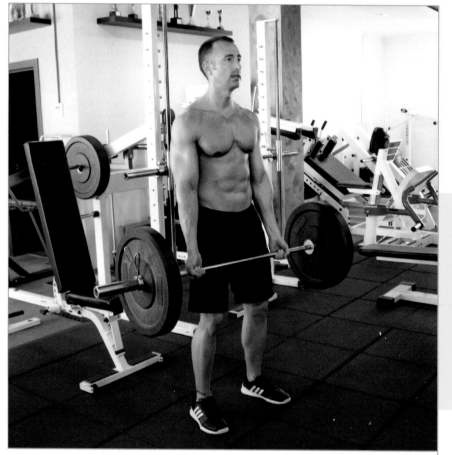

If a competitive bodybuilder is training his biceps, executing 1 series of 6 repetitions of a curl, lifting a lemon, they will obviously not experience any improvement. Nonetheless, if they complete 32 series of 18 repetitions each of a curl with a bar, lifting 50 kg, they will probably hurt themselves or spend 15 days without being able to move their arms. The low effort does not stimulate and the excessive effort injures them, so that they must find the right point.

The demands of excessive training will ruin any athlete's season

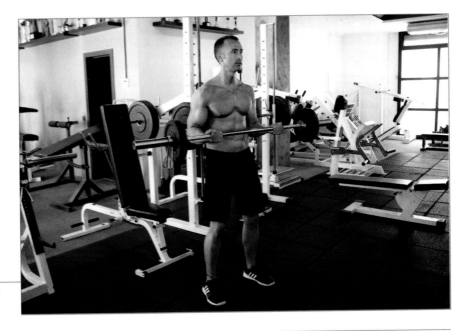

A healthy individual has internal balance, or homeostasis, which we picture in the next graphic as a straight line. A stringing together of insufficient stimuli does not cause any change in their condition, but always returns them to the original line of equilibrium.

Insufficient training loads do not result in any improvement.

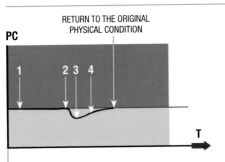

The stimulus does not lead to improvements.

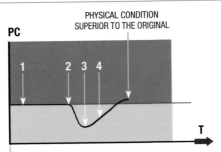

Sufficient stimulus causes improvements in the athlete's physical condition.

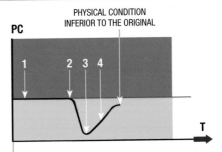

Excessive stimuli worsen the physical condition of the athlete.

PC: Physical condition.
T: Time.
1: Initial physical condition
2: Application of the training load
3: Decrease in the physical condition related to the load
4: Recovery

Practical Recommendation: since the training load is determined by volume and intensity, here is an example of how to apply each one of these parameters.

Volume: according to scientific evidence, as a function of the individual, the training volume that generates the greatest benefits in muscle gain for the new athlete is between 3 and 8 series; each one of them should include between 6 and 12 repetitions, and one must consider small variations in this number of repetitions from time to time. Advanced athletes may require a higher training volume.

The speed of execution of each repetition that evidences the greatest benefits swings between 1 and 6 seconds, with the positive phase of the exercise being the quicker phase than the negative. This time under pressure produces sufficient metabolic stress (perceived by the athlete as swelling, congestion or burning), one of the key factors for muscular hypertrophy.

Intensity: the intensity of the work must be high; completing a series of between 6 and 12 repetitions must result in muscle failure, which makes it possible to recruit the maximum number of fibers, providing that the mechanical tension (another key factor for hypertrophy) is high.

Principle of overcompensation

When we subject our body to stress, the body tends to recover until it reaches a higher level than the one it had before receiving the stimulus. When we subject it to a training load, it is not just a case of returning to its original form, but rather it is trying to exceed this form for the purpose of being better prepared to deal with a next training effort. This phenomenon is known as overcompensation.

This principle is closely tied to that of overload, since in order for overcompensation to occur, the stimulus must be sufficient and not too easy or excessive. It is the body's mechanism for dealing with successive training loads, each time under better conditions. It is also related to the principle of continuity, the 4th on the list, which is shown here.

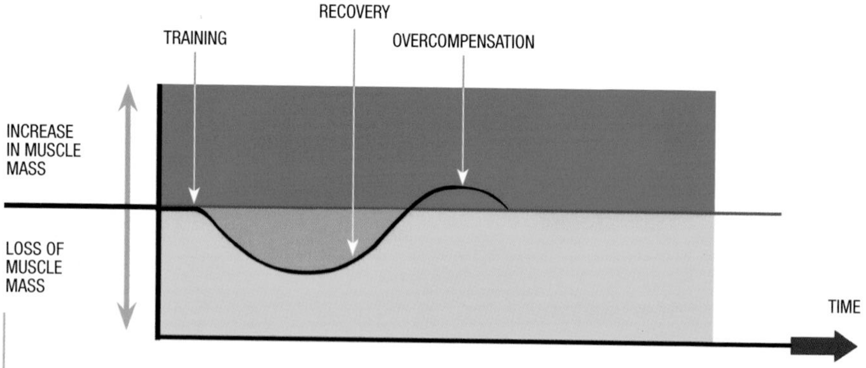

The body performs like the individual; thus, if we go to a university exam without having first studied, it is likely that we will fail. Before going to the re-test, we will study and improve our preparation in order to take the test again with assurance of passing. The body works the same way; it receives a stimulus and prepares to confront the next one with greater assurance.

Measurable improvements in an athlete's performance do not occur after a one-time training session, since the process of overcompensation is reduced and only the stringing together of these processes will reveal obvious improvement.

RECOVERY

TRAINING   OVERCOMPENSATION

INCREASE
IN MUSCLE
MASS

LOSS OF
MUSCLE
MASS

TIME

After the stimulus, there is a momentary drop in performance and then recovery, and finally, recovery extends until the athlete achieves a somewhat higher performance level than their original level.

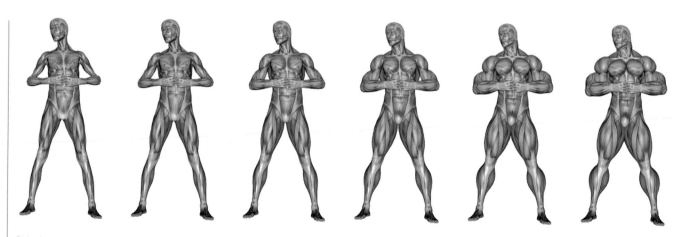

Stringing together the processes of overcompensation will produce physical improvements and performance in the individual.

Principle of Continuity

Training must be repeated on a schedule and the preparation process must be continuous so that adaptations will be progressive and significant. If you train once and do not train again in the next three weeks, this improvement from overcompensation will be diluted over time and you will return to your original state. Improvement requires continuous and thorough practice so that increments in performance will be cumulative.

This principle is difficult for the majority of new athletes to follow, since it is hard to train day after day without seeing immediate results, and many times, this is the reason for a quick abandonment of the activity. In reality, results appear after months of hard training and disappear in a few weeks inactivity. This is why there is greater emphasis on the importance of consistency for progress and maintenance.

The body must economize resources and rid itself of the things that it does not need, or those that cause it to expend energy. Thus, a very muscular athlete who will maintain their powerful muscles while their body needs to conserve them, will lift weights several times per week. When physical activity ceases, these rapidly decrease, because they require a high energy expenditure and there is no activity to justify maintaining them.

The same thing happens when we put on a cast and immobilize a leg for several weeks. When the cast is taken off, this leg has less muscle mass than the other one, due to the period of inactivity.

Successive training loads generate a progressive improvement in performance

PHYSICAL CONDITION

LOAD 1 LOAD 2 LOAD 3 IMPROVEMENT

TIME

Practical recommendation: recommended training frequencies for the same muscle are two to three times per week, with various muscle groups being able to be trained in a single session. Nonetheless, advanced athletes who use divided routines are used to working each muscle group only once per week and their training volume is higher.

*Only those athletes who are able to persist and string together training sessions will achieve outstanding results.
In addition, they must also maintain appropriate feeding and rest routines for months or years.*

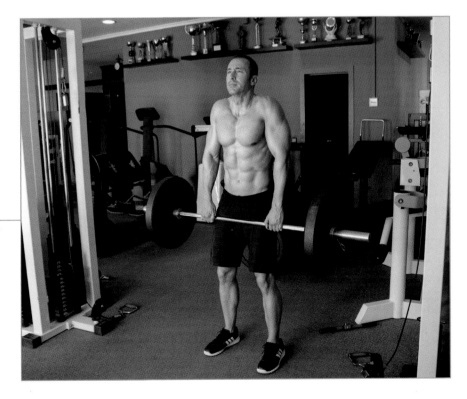

Principle of progression

Training loads must be increased periodically in order to avoid any stagnation in the athlete's progression. If you apply the same training load indefinitely, you will only obtain results for a limited time. Once you have adapted to this work load, your improvement will stop and you will enter into a stagnation phase. In order to keep improving, you will have to keep increasing the stimulus applied as your physical condition improves.

This work load could be increased by acting on one of the two factors that determine it (volume and intensity), or on both of them at the same time and always progressively, in small increments. The usual approach is to act on intensity. In general, this means modifying the weight by absolute values, then continuing with the same percentage of 1RM.

Another way to vary the work load is to modify the volume. In order to do this, add series or exercises to your usual routine.

A new athlete can begin performing an exercise with a low weight, they must work at 80% of their 1RM in order to do so. As the training sessions follow each other and become stronger, this same weight every time assumes some lower percentage of their 1RM. For this reason, they must continue to increase the total weight with which they are working, so that it continues to use 80% of their 1 RM and they continue to work at a sufficient intensity..

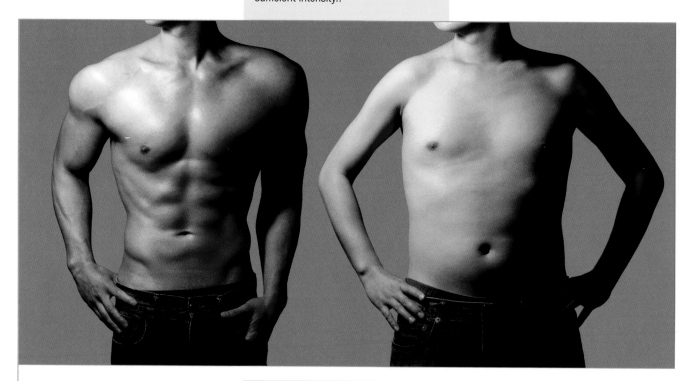

The same athlete before and after following a strength training routine for one year and a half. It is obvious that the resistances with which they were training at the beginning and those that they use now, must be different.

Practical recommendation: in order to work in a sufficient range of intensities, they must arrive at muscle failure between the repetition 6 and 12. If it is impossible to reach 6 consecutive repetitions, it is likely that they are working too intensely. If, on the other hand, they exceed 12 repetitions easily, they should add difficulty to the exercise.

Progression is not always linear, since after arriving at a determined level, it is easy to stagnate. Alternating periods of greater training loads and others with smaller loads has proven to be effective at these times.

Principle of recovery

Any effort or physical exertion requires a later rest and recovery period, for the purpose of producing positive adaptations in performance. Namely, after applying a training load, the body needs a determined recovery time so that it can complete the process of overcompensation.

This principle has a simple logic and is related to the maxim that more is not always better. Likewise, more often is not always better.

Not allowing sufficient time between training sessions or training sessions for the same muscle group results in over training, chronic fatigue, a drop in performance, pains, recurring injuries, decrease in defenses, etc.

Likewise, allowing for long rest periods between training sessions will result in the dissipation of performance improvements, since, as we recall, the body tends to economize resources.

A marathon athlete can train with runs of 20-30 km and obtain good results. However, if they run 3 sessions of 20 km per day, without any recovery time, the result will be catastrophic.

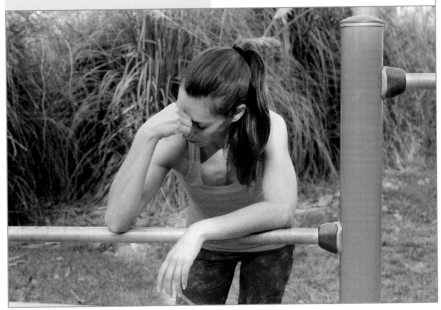

Lack of sufficient rest for recovery will result in chronic fatigue and a decrease in performance.

Not allowing for sufficient rest between sessions will have the immediate consequence of a worsening physical condition.

1: Application of load 1.
2: Application of load 2.
3: Application of load 3.
3: Application of load 4.

Excessive rest will result in the achieved adaptations being lost.

1: Application of load 1.
2: Optimal moment for the application of a new load.
3: Loss of the adaptation and return to original condition.
4: Application of load 2.
5: Application of load 3.

Practical recommendation: for the recommended training loads, it is a good idea to allow time between training sessions for the same muscle group of between 48 and 72 hours. Advanced athletes who use greater training loads must continue to increase rest periods up to a maximum of 6 -7 days. It is also important to leave pauses between series. For hypertrophy training, these times swing between 60 and 120 seconds with the goal of finding a balance between metabolic stress and mechanical tension.

INCREASE IN PERFORMANCE

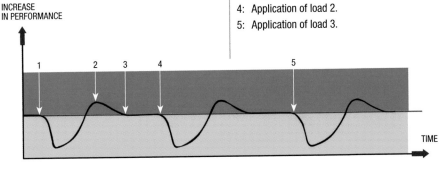

Principle of variety

Introducing changes and variations into your repertory of exercises, intensity, volume and other training parameters, is a key factor in nearing the maximum performance potential of an athlete. Within the general parameters of a discipline, introducing small variations in the applied stimuli will succeed in preventing your body from completely adapting to an unvarying routine and, therefore, will continue its improvement.

If you always use the same exercises, which include an equal number of series, repetitions, pause times and duration of repetitions, you will reach a point where your body becomes accustomed to this repetitive process, causing the improvement to stop.

Introducing small changes into the exercises, in the work angles, times under tension, etc., will provide sufficient variation so that you will never be completely adapted to the stimulus, and in addition, will avoid monotony and lack of motivation.

Introduce regular changes into your training in order to not lose sight of your objective and of the basic parameters for obtaining improvements in a specific discipline.

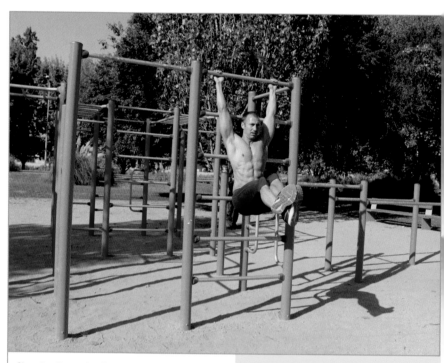

The introduction of periodic changes in inclination, movement, grips, speed, position and other variations of the different exercises enables us to continue effective growth stimuli to the muscles.

Changing the angle of execution of a crunch will introduce a small variation which will bring you benefits.

Practical recommendation: new athletes will need some time to internalize the motor patterns of certain exercises and master their techniques, in order to develop all of their ability in executing them. For this reason, once your training exercises are included, these should be maintained between 4 and 8 weeks before introducing changes. On the other hand, advanced athletes who have internalized the technique and are able to perfectly master it, even after months of not practicing, will be able to vary their routines with greater frequency, making the most of the principle of variety. It should be recalled that, even though it is a good idea to work with maximum ranges of movement or articulator amplitude (ROM), here, it is also possible to introduce variations in angles and repetitions from time to time.

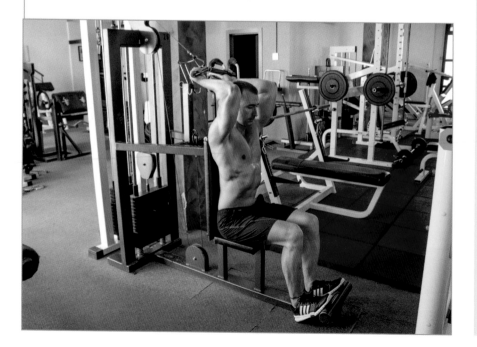

Principle of individualization

General training programs are often applied to a large number of very different athletes in gyms. This is not necessarily something negative, since a typical training program will produce more or less positive results in 90% of such athletes, especially if they are new athletes.

When an athlete of middle or advanced ability nears his improvement ceiling, the details begin to take on more importance so training should therefore be adjusted to his individual response. Thus, it can be that two partners who train together, after 3 years of almost identical work, will begin to require individual adaptations. It may be that one of them recovers from a leg training session in 48 hours and, nonetheless, the other one requires 72 hours, or even that one of them reacts to training sessions of 6 series per muscle group, and the other obtains better results with 8-9 series. The same is true for the number and speed of execution of the repetitions in each series or of the pauses between series.

Practical recommendation: everyone can start by executing typical routines. Nonetheless, as your level improves, you will have to continue adjusting the training to the individual characteristics of each person in order to be able to continue improving. Careful observation of one's own evolution, as well as experimentation and the application of periodic changes, are the best system for discovering what does and does not work.

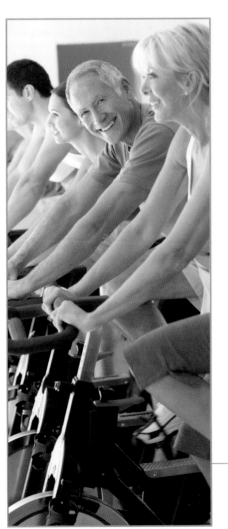

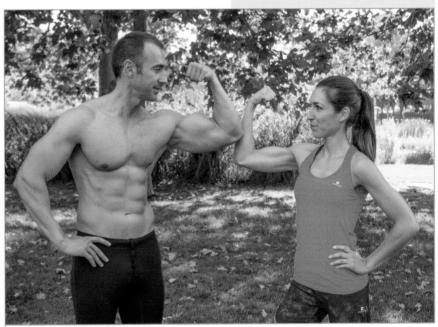

Different individuals need different types of training to advance.

Typical programs can produce relatively good results in the majority of athletes in the first stages of training.

Principle of diminishing returns

Regardless of how basic the experience and level of the athlete is, improvements and quicker results will be obtained through successive training sessions. As your physical condition and performance improve, your rate of improvement will slow down. The closer this rate gets to its maximum potential, the more difficult it will be to continue improving.

Thus, it may be that you have a good memory of a training routine, because you obtained magnificent results when you started it. Now, with much greater muscular development, you will use more advanced training routines and techniques and, even so, your increase in muscle mass will be less, and improvements will only happen intermittently.

It may even happen that you experience periods of stagnation or that your physical condition temporarily worsens. This is normal when performance is high and is reaching a level that is close to your maximum genetic potential. For this reason, it is a good idea for variations in your training style, and routine planning to become habitual.

You must aspire to get as close to your maximum potential as possible, but this is a moving target which is impossible to determine, so that you must not lose the goal of improving, including during times when you are not experiencing advances. You will be a better athlete if you develop the ability to persist, even when the expectations are hard to define.

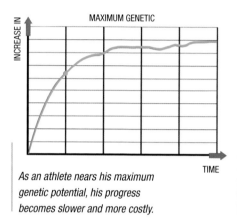

As an athlete nears his maximum genetic potential, his progress becomes slower and more costly.

Practical recommendation: when, despite hard training, diet and rest, you find that you have stagnated, or even lessened in your performance, the best options are to introduce variety or to take a break. The latter option consists of not training for 1-2 weeks, since you may need to disconnect from training sessions, or give your body some marginal rest days for a deep recovery.

The most advanced athletes will also be those who encounter the most difficulties in continuing to improve.

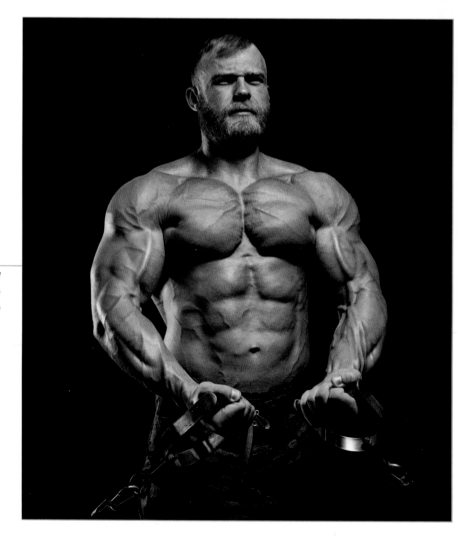

Important data review

Other than the PRINCIPLES OF TRAINING, here are three basic elements that every strength training athlete must consider when designing their training sessions. These elements are mechanical tension, muscle damage and metabolic stress. Following, we recall a series of practical recommendations to get the greatest benefit out of each of them.

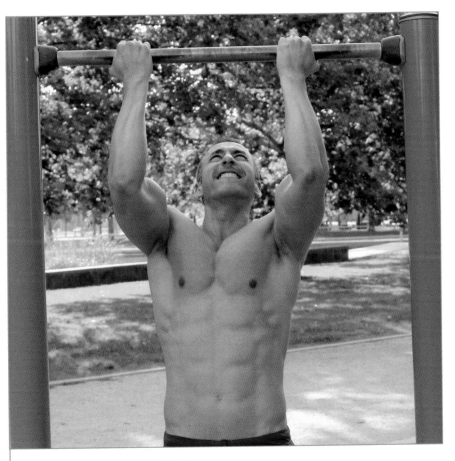

Mechanical tension is an important factor for muscle growth and involves working at high intensities.

MECHANICAL TENSION

Mechanical tension is generated as a result of resistance work and is believed to be the principal factor of inducing muscular hypertrophy. The degree of hypertrophic response to mechanical tension is determined by the duration and intensity of its application. Therefore, you must find a balance between execution time and applied resistance. In order to maximize your progression in relation to mechanical tension:

• Use resistances that round to .80% 1 RM.

• Avoid very short rests between series, or very long series, because these will work against managing heavy weights and the mechanical tension factor will lose efficacy.

• Try to reach muscle failure, except during recovery steps. High intensity and series that exceed 25 seconds will enable you to recruit a greater number of fibers.

MUSCLE DAMAGE

As a result of working against high resistances, the muscles break down. Muscle tissue is damaged due to training, which is normal, and drives the hypertrophic response, especially in advanced athletes. In order to take advantage of this factor, you should consider that:

• Muscle damage as a consequence of exercise promotes the recovery and strengthening of the tissue. Nonetheless, you should rest between training sessions of the same muscle group, for no less than 48-72 hours, or more, in advanced athletes who use higher training loads.

• Excessive muscle damage will have a negative effect on progress. Avoid endless or excessive training sessions.

The three elements associated with a muscular hypertrophy reaction are:

METABOLIC STRESS

This results from muscle work, especially against resistance, which is executed in short periods of time (the time of one series) and requires a high energy contribution. This energy flow is contributed by an anaerobic glycolysis process that generates specific byproducts, which accumulate in the muscle. This environment produces a notable anabolic response, especially if these sub-products do not efficiently evacuate from the blood stream, due to muscular congestion, which constricts the blood vessels and makes return circulation more difficult. In order to take advantage of this factor, it is a good idea:

• To execute various series for one muscle group, between 3 and 8, or more, for advanced athletes.

• Each repetition must last from 1 to 6 seconds, with the negative phase being slower than the positive phase.

• Rests between series should not be very long (60-120 seconds).

Plan your own routines

There are a thousand ways to plan training routines, with exercises available in lines, grids, written form only, with drawings, photos or even with videos showing you how to execute them. The majority of routines prepared by athletes themselves and not at specialized centers, are only a sheet of paper with handwritten notes.

Finally, the important thing is the contents of the plan and the deliberation and consideration with which the plan was prepared. Even if the content is attractive, this has absolutely nothing to do with its quality and suitability.

In general, programs must be distributed over several days of training and each one should prioritize one or more muscles. If your program takes into account that you will work each muscle at least twice a week, you will have to exercise a number of muscles during each session. This does not mean that you may perform an exercise for a muscle group, then begin with another group and after, return to the first to do the second exercise. This does not make any sense, because it involves cutting the work process in half, in order to later go back to it, stopping a series of processes that lead to optimum performance and growth stimulation. You can, however, work two muscle groups simultaneously, if you alternate between them.

An athlete may execute a series of parallel inclined dips for the chest, and, during the rest, do pull-ups, and repeat the process for successive series, taking advantage of the recovery pause for one group of muscles to work on the other group.

The visually most attractive routine will almost never be the best, especially if it is an example routine.

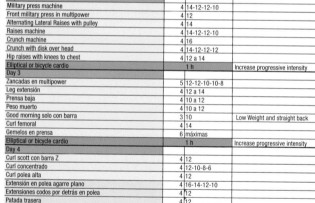

		Instruction
		Add weight progressively
		Do not open much (shoulders close)
		Add weight progressively
Cross Pulleys	4	16-14-14-12	
Elliptical or bicycle cardio	1 h		Increase progressive intensity
Day 2			
Military press machine	4	14-12-12-10	
Front military press in multipower	4	12	
Alternating Lateral Raises with pulley	4	14	
Raises machine	4	14-12-12-10	
Crunch machine	4	16	
Crunch with disk over head	4	14-12-12-12	
Hip raises with knees to chest	4	12 a 14	
Elliptical or bicycle cardio	1 h		Increase progressive intensity
Day 3			
Zancadas en multipower	5	12-12-10-10-8	
Leg extensión	4	12 a 14	
Prensa baja	4	10 a 12	
Peso muerto	4	10 a 12	
Good morning solo con barra	3	10	Low Weight and straight back
Curl femoral	4	14	
Gemelos en prensa	6	máximas	
Elliptical or bicycle cardio	1 h		Increase progressive intensity
Day 4			
Curl scott con barra Z	4	12	
Curl concentrado	4	12-10-8-6	
Curl polea alta	4	12	
Extensión en polea agarre plano	4	16-14-12-10	
Extensiones codos por detrás en polea	4	12	
Patada trasera	4	12	

Using the rest between series for one muscle group to work on another is a good, time-saving method.

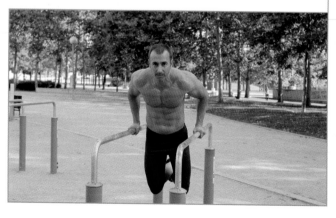

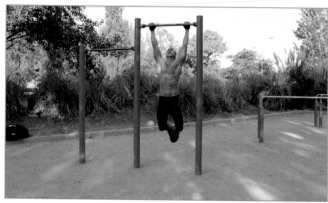

Alternating series with different muscles saves time and is highly advisable if you are working opposing muscles. You should not do alternating series to work one muscle and another that was used in the same exercise as the first.

For example, if you are working the latissimus dorsi, never combine it with biceps exercises, since the majority of back exercises involve the participation of the biceps, and they will not recover either for their own series or to assist in back series. The same is true with the chest and triceps, or with the chest and shoulders.

MONDAY/DAY 1:
- Chest   4 x 12 – 10-8-8
  - Flies with towels   3 x 12
  - Deep push-ups w/jumps
- Back   4 x 14 -12-12-10
  - Suspended row   3 x 12
  - Pull-ups
- Abdominals   4 x 12
  - Vertical arm crunch   3 x 12 -10-10
  - Inclined hip raises

TUESDAY/DAY 2:
- Shoulders   4 x 16 -14-12-12
  - Lateral raises   3 x 12 -10-8
  - Front press
- Triceps   4 x 12 -12-10-10
  - Diamond push-ups   3 x 10 -8-6
  - Dips
- Biceps   4 x 12
  - Auto-resistance curl w/foot   3 x 12
  - Suspended curls

WEDNESDAY/DAY 3
- Quadriceps....

If you work the triceps and then the chest, you will not be able to do pushing exercises for the chest since the triceps are already fatigued.

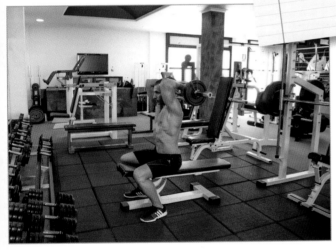

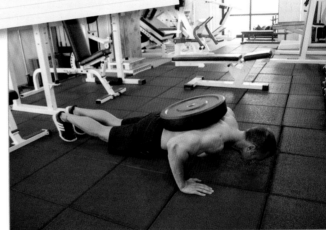

In the same way, if, in order to train a large muscle, you include mono-articular and bi-articular exercises, such as flies or flexions, do the mono-articular exercises first, so that the most powerful muscle (pectoralis major) is fatigued first, and you will prevent the weaker muscle (brachial triceps) from being a limiting factor in the bi-articular exercise.

We recommend that you plan your training week taking these issues into account:
- Number of days or sessions of training.
- Muscle groups per session, and their organization.
- Exercises to perform and the order for their performance.
- Number of series per exercise and number of repetitions per series.
- Always include a few minutes for general warm-up before beginning, and one or two series of high repetitions and low resistance specific warm-up for each muscle group. It is not necessary to show this in your written plan.

If you train the triceps and then go to the chest, it will be difficult for the triceps to work with the chest muscles in exercises that push the chest, since they are already fatigued. The same happens when you train the biceps and then the back.

Appropriate diet

A proper diet is the athlete's best ally. The key factor is to adapt diet to your lifestyle and the type of training you are doing. Nutritional requirements of athletes, or those who are subject to greater than average wear and tear, are very different from those of a sedentary person, and it is important to adapt them to the physical activity of the individual and his or her performance goals.

The human body needs to ingest three macronutrients in high quantities every day: proteins, carbohydrates and lipids or fats. The quantities, type and combination of these in the different meals of the day are determinants for the growth of muscle mass.

PROTEINS

Each gram of protein contains 4 kcal and yet, the body "prefers" carbohydrates and fats as sources of energy. However, protein has a very important function, especially for hypertrophy athletes: it is the structural function. It is impossible to grow and build new tissue without a sufficient amount of proteins. Nonetheless, proteins also have other functions, for example, in hormonal regulation, defenses, chemical reactions, transport and signaling in our body.

Proteins are molecules comprised of amino acids, and their work in building

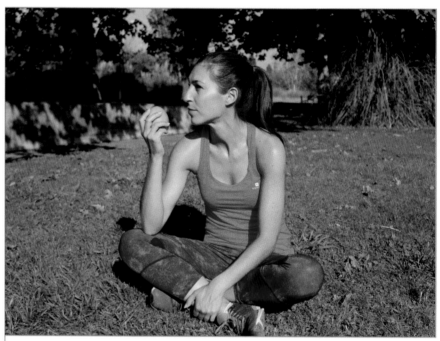

There is a series of parameters you must meet in order to achieve a healthy diet.

Essential amino acids	Non-essential amino acids
Isoleucine	Alanine
Leucine	Arginine
Lysine	Asparagine
Methionine	Aspartic Acid
Phenylalanine	Cystenine
Treonine	Glutamic Acid
Tryptophan	Clycine
Valine	Proline
Histidine	Serine
	Tyrosine
	Glutamine

muscle tissue is determined by their ability to provide these amino acids to the proteins that build body tissues among these muscles. There are hundreds of amino acids, but barely 20 participate in these processes, so we must find ways of obtaining them.

There are 9 essential amino acids, which the body cannot synthesize and must be obtained through diet. On the other hand, the non-essential ones are those that the body can synthesize, and does not need to ingest, unless it requires a greater quantity than the body is capable of synthesizing.

It is not enough to ingest protein. You must also consider the amount and quality of the protein ingested, as well as its distribution throughout the day.

Quality

The 9 essential amino acids that our body cannot synthesize, and must therefore ingest, are not present in all proteins. Those of animal origin, except for any exception, are very complete, that is, they contain all of the essential amino acids. On the other hand, plant proteins lack some of these, so are incomplete.

If you choose to obtain proteins by a supplement, apply the same parameters as for the rest of your meals. The origin of the protein will determine whether it is or is not complete.

Quantity

The recommended daily amount of protein for a sedentary person is between 0.8 and 1 gram per kilogram of weight per day. Those who engage in physical activity must meet greater needs.

It is estimated that a bodybuilding athlete must consume between 1.7 and 2.4 grams per kilogram of weight per day in order to meet her specific needs as an athlete and continue developing her muscles. Nonetheless, there are specific factors that influence the increase or decrease in protein needs.

Proteins of animal origin contain all of the essential amino acids.

Practical recommendation: try to ensure that the protein portion of each of your meals is of animal origin, which includes milk products and eggs. Foods of plant origin do not have all of the essential amino acids, although they can be combined so as to complement each other, which will require prior planning.

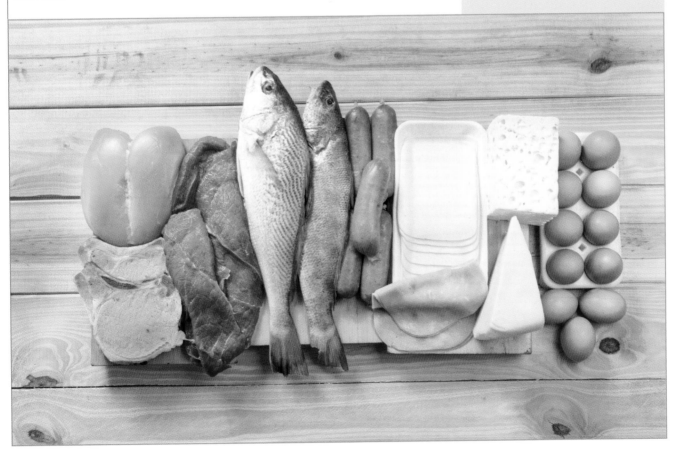

Young athletes will have sufficient protein for maintenance in the lowest rank of the cited values, but as the years pass, the body's use of protein may become less efficient so that older athletes must use the quantities cited in the highest of the recommended ranges.

It is important to also highlight that experienced athletes have, over time, adapted their regular bodybuilding activities and, as a result, their use of protein may be slightly more efficient leading to them only requiring lower amounts.

Finally, athletes who consume a diet low in carbohydrates in order to reduce their level of body fat, need to approach 3 grams per kilogram of body weight in order to minimize the loss of muscle mass.

Have five light and balanced meals each day, since this will provide you with what you need, when you need it.

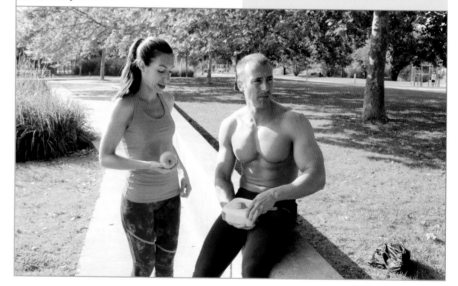

Practical recommendation: eat every 3 to 4 hours, in reasonable amounts and provide the body with an adequate dose of all of the macronutrients that you need at each meal until you have had five light meals each day.

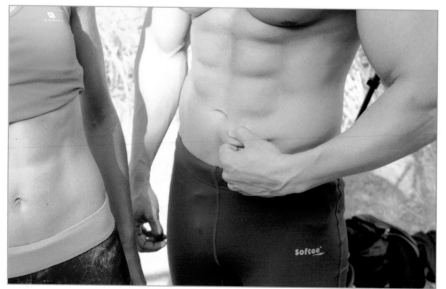

In phases of hypo-caloric diet in order to reduce the level of body fat, the ingestion of protein will be a little higher.

Frequency

The use of protein is more efficient if we distribute its consumption throughout the diet and every few hours; this will guarantee a continuous input to meet the recovery needs of the body.

After a training session, recovery is continuous and progressive for many hours, so it is not enough to have a large portion of protein after exercise. It must be eaten every few hours. This is not a special feature of protein, and must be applied to the other macronutrients. A number of small portions distributed throughout the day will be more efficient than one or two large portions at the principal meals.

CARBOHYDRATES

Carbohydrates, along with proteins, have 4 kcal per gram, with the difference being that their principal function is to provide energy. They provide energy for daily activities and in a very significant way, for bodybuilding training sessions.

A diet low in carbohydrates can substantially reduce an athlete's performance, and he may feel weakness and fatigue well before his expectation. Therefore, we recommend having an adequate amount of carbohydrates in each of the five daily meals in order to achieve maximum performance.

Despite this, carbohydrates may affect the body differently. For example, ingesting 10 grams of carbohydrates in the form of whole wheat bread is not the same as ingesting them as refined sugar.

The Glycemic Index

The glycemic index measures the effect of consuming a food, using blood sugar levels and, finally, using the insulin response it causes. The quantity and structure of the carbohydrates in the food does not completely determine it, but it is a factor which must be considered. If we ingest a food that raises blood sugar a great deal, and very suddenly, we will cause insulin levels, the function of which is to enable this blood glucose to move into the cells in order to meet their energy needs, to be out of control until these blood sugar levels return to normal.

The problem arises when the energy input is much greater than the energy needs of these cells at the moment. All of this unused energy must be stored, and is done so through the forming of fat.

Choose foods that are rich in carbohydrates that are more adapted to each moment, prioritizing those with a low GI, except at those times when there are higher energy needs.

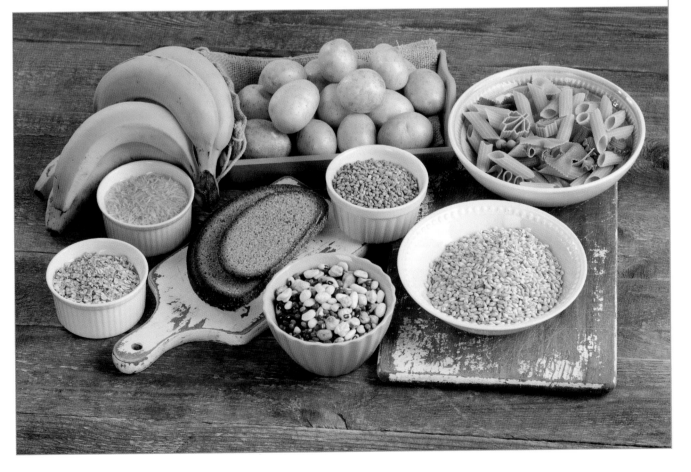

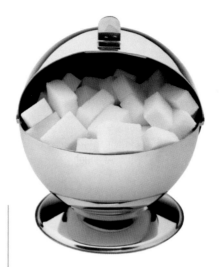

For this reason, foods with a high GI, such as sugar, will cause you to gain weight more easily than those with a lower GI, such as black bread, even if you ingest the same number of grams of carbohydrates.

On the other hand, foods with a low glycemic index make it possible for blood glucose levels to be maintained or to rise slowly and gradually over a longer period of time. Thus, insulin levels will remain more stable and energy will be delivered to the cells in a constant and regulated form. This continuous energy stream, with its low flow rate, will deliver this fuel to the cells as the cells consume it, thus avoiding any excess being stored in the form of fat in adipose tissue.

However, on rare occasions, it will be appropriate to consume foods with a high GI level. For example, after an exhausting training session during which muscular glycogen deposits have been very diminished and, above all, if you are going to train again during the same day, you could consume some food with a high GI level such as boiled potato or quick-cook white rice, banana or sweet potato. This will raise insulin levels above where they are at present due to the physical activity and will replenish your muscle glycogen reserves quickly. If, in addition, you add a source of protein, the anabolic environment will be perfect to promote a better and quicker recovery.

Foods with a high GI create body fat more easily.

Practical recommendation: eat carbohydrates at every meal, but not in excess. Choose those that have a lower GI, such as whole grain cereals and their derivatives with whole grain flours.

Foods with a high GI should be reserved for very rare treats and for drinking immediately after very demanding training sessions.

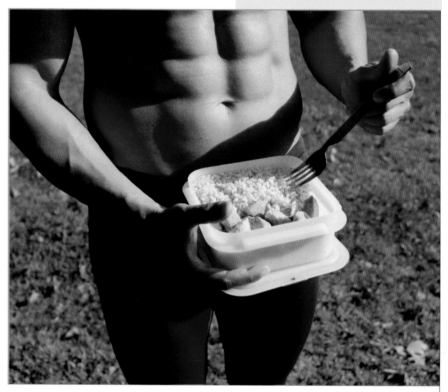

It is appropriate to eat carbohydrates and protein after training in order to improve recovery.

FATS

Lipids, or fats, have 9 kcal per gram, which implies an energy contribution that is much greater in quantity, although not necessarily in availability, than that of proteins and carbohydrates. They play an important role as energy reserves, and they also function to insulate and protect our bodies and internal organs, and even help to transport some vitamins in the blood flow and storage. An appropriate diet does not leave out fats, but they should only be consumed within reason. Three different types of fat must be distinguished.

Saturated Fats

In general, these are of animal origin and are solid at room temperature, such as butter, lard and cream. Some are of plant origin, such as palm oil. These fats are not recommended and should be avoided, too, because they will cause you to gain weight and, long term, will increase the risk of suffering from metabolic and cardiovascular disease. Medium chain triglycerides, or MCTs, such as coconut oil, are an exception, because they metabolize differently and their moderate consumption may be advisable.

Monounsaturated fats

These are often of plant origin and are liquid at room temperature. Although it is not a good idea to abuse these fats, they are healthy and remain stable when exposed to heat, due to which, to fry a food, it is better to use a monounsaturated fat such as olive oil.

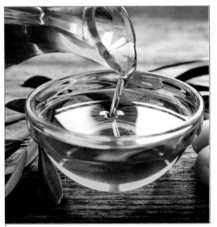

Olive oil,
monounsaturated fat

Sunflower oil,
polyunsaturated. fat.

Polyunsaturated fat

These are found in plant and animal foods and are liquid at room temperature. These are also considered to be healthy fats. Omega 3 and 6 fatty acids reduce levels of LDL cholesterol and levels of saturated fats in the body, in addition to protecting the cardiovascular system.

They are better for you, but are not very resistant to heat, so a sunflower oil will be appropriate for dressing a salad but not for frying foods.

Practical recommendation: eat fats daily because they are necessary to the proper functioning of the body. Choose polyunsaturated fats, such as sunflower oil, to eat uncooked, and monounsaturated fats such as olive oil when cooking with heat, especially with fried foods. Avoid regular consumption of saturated fats, with the occasional exception of the MCTs.

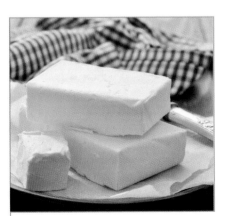

Butter, saturated fat

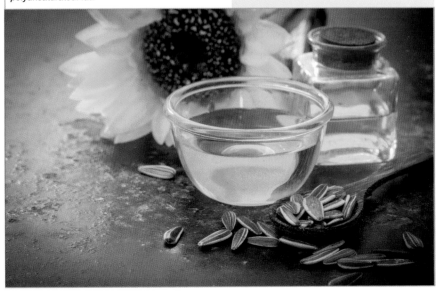

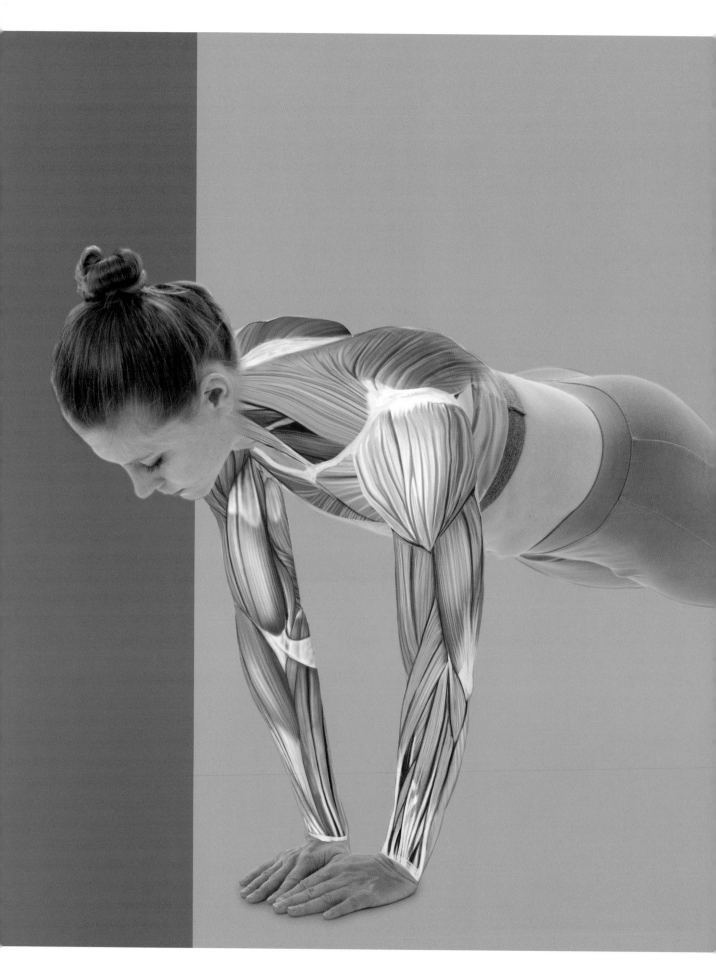

Exercises

Next, we will show you some exercises you can do without any equipment, or with non-specialized equipment, to strengthen your muscles. This is obviously a small sample of the great variety of existing exercises. It is a selection that you can use to work all muscle groups, including variations of differing difficulty so that any exerciser, regardless of your level, will find exercises that are suited to your training routine, including modifications of these exercises which are adapted to your progress. It is up to each person to choose the options most aligned with his or her physical and material abilities. Remember, something that works for one individual may have a different effect on another.

We also invite you to modify the exercises that appear here, and to design new ones that comply with basic safety parameters. The exerciser who understands the function of each muscle and its specificities, as well as the basic principles of muscle training will be the one suited to designing his own routines, and modifying them periodically, depending on his or her needs and responses to training. You will be able to observe, test, select, modify and adapt the exercises and training routines critically and with the self-knowledge that only you, as the exerciser, have.

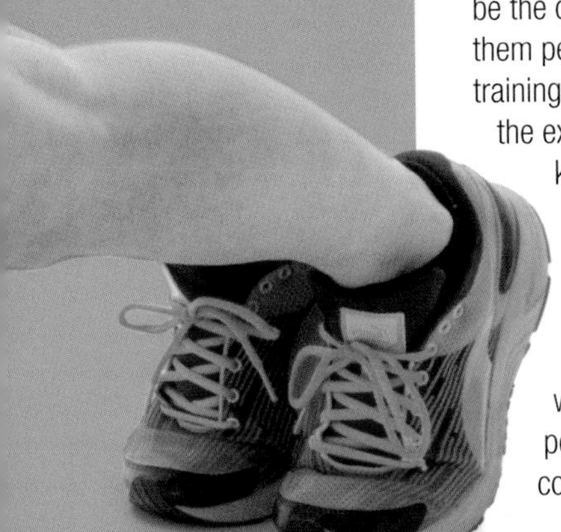

Try to comply with general training principles and use variety as a means to escape boredom and stagnation. When you believe you are ready to work on your own, review the exercises we are showing and after a while, it will be worthwhile to record and implement those which you have perhaps forgotten, and limit yourself to those which, due to convenience or habit, have become essential to your sessions.

01 Push-Ups

This is one of the best-known exercises in training, using only bodyweight. It has been used for decades by various groups and its many variations make it possible to vary its degree of difficulty.

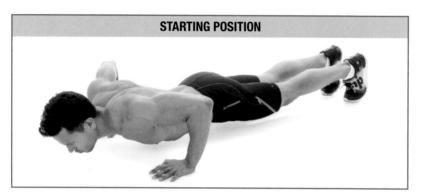

STARTING POSITION

MUSCULAR INTENSITY

+

7

−

Execution

Lie face down, with the palms of your hands on the ground, so that they are at either side of your chest, but without touching it. Also push your toes into the ground and keep your back and legs straight, keeping your body parallel to the ground and as close as possible to the ground, without touching it. From this position, straighten your elbows and raise your body so that your chest moves away from the ground.

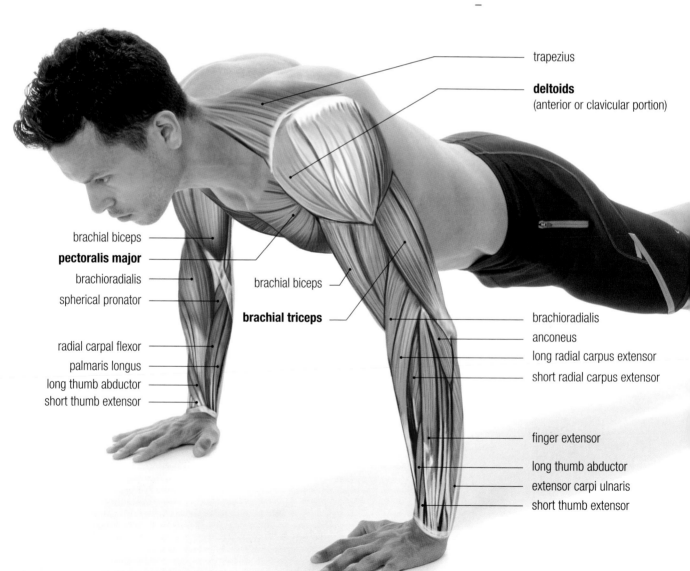

trapezius

deltoids
(anterior or clavicular portion)

brachial biceps

pectoralis major

brachioradialis

spherical pronator

brachial biceps

brachial triceps

radial carpal flexor

palmaris longus

long thumb abductor

short thumb extensor

brachioradialis

anconeus

long radial carpus extensor

short radial carpus extensor

finger extensor

long thumb abductor

extensor carpi ulnaris

short thumb extensor

ALTERNATIVE EXERCISES 01

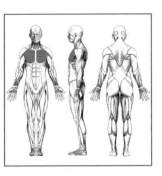

Technical considerations

■ Your trunk and lower extremities must be in perfect alignment.

■ Limit the movement of your elbows and shoulders.

■ Lower yourself as far as possible without using the ground to support your weight.

■ Easier variation

If a normal push-up is very difficult for you to execute, instead of pushing your toes into the ground for support, try supporting yourself on your knees, preferably on a mat. This exercise will make it possible for you to work at a lower intensity until you are able to do traditional push-ups.

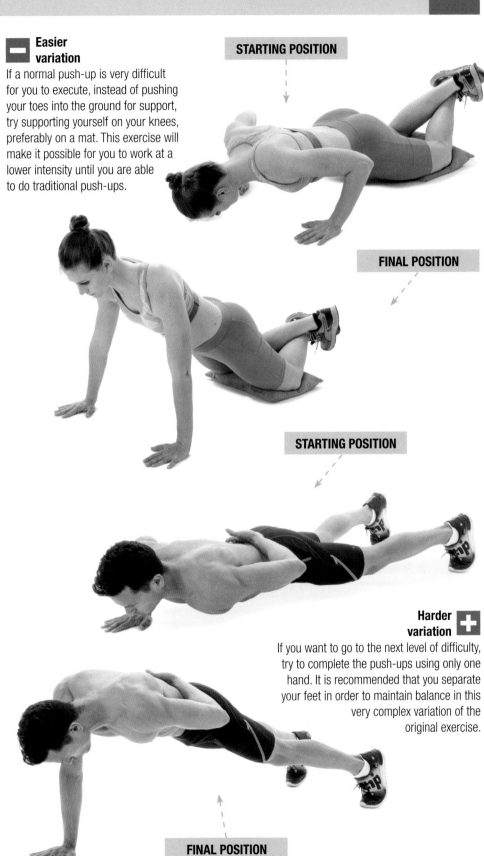

STARTING POSITION

FINAL POSITION

STARTING POSITION

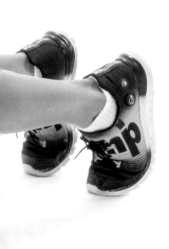

Harder ⊞ variation

If you want to go to the next level of difficulty, try to complete the push-ups using only one hand. It is recommended that you separate your feet in order to maintain balance in this very complex variation of the original exercise.

FINAL POSITION

02 | Suspension Push-Ups

$\mathbf{S}$uspension devices, which have become very popular in recent years, are a good complement for our exercises and provide variety. Although they are not very expensive, we can still make our own devices for an even lower cost. Nylon belts for fastening loads are a cheap, tough, and durable alternative and are able to support loads above 100 kg.

+

9

MUSCULAR INTENSITY

−

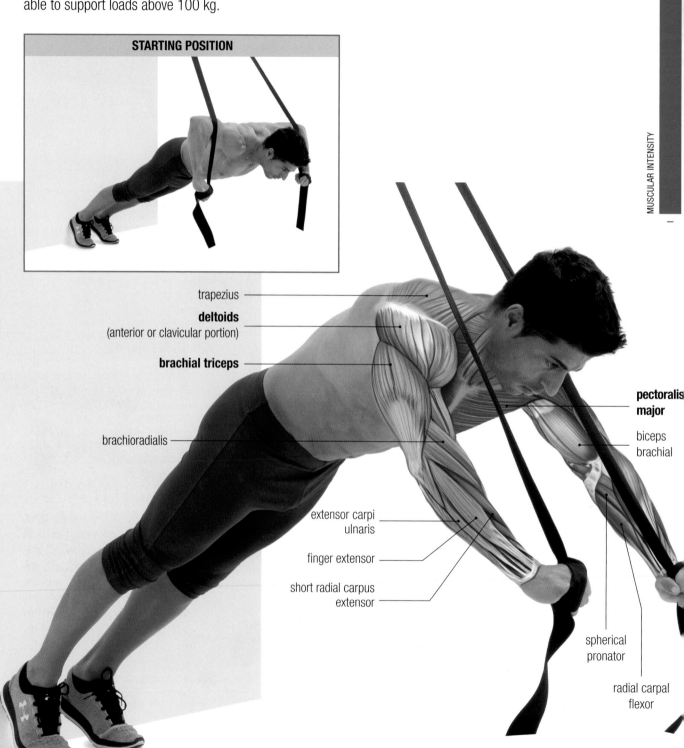

STARTING POSITION

trapezius

deltoids
(anterior or clavicular portion)

brachial triceps

brachioradialis

pectoralis major

biceps brachial

extensor carpi ulnaris

finger extensor

short radial carpus extensor

spherical pronator

radial carpal flexor

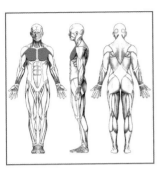

Execution

Set the suspension training belt or device for elevated support and hold one end with each hand.

Extend your elbows so that the palms of your hands are in front of you and continue to lean down so that the belt is supporting part of your weight. Flex your elbows as if you were doing a push-up on the ground and then extend them again.

Technical considerations

- The belt does not provide the same stability as the ground, so in addition to overcoming your weight, you must overcome its instability.

- Keep your trunk and thighs aligned.

- The greater the angle, the greater the difficulty.

STARTING POSITION

Easier variation

In order to begin working the technique of the principal exercise, particularly if you are not accustomed to suspension training, you can perform this alternative for which the inclination of the body is minimal. The resistance is noticeably reduced, but you will be able to experiment with support with the instability of belts.

FINAL POSITION

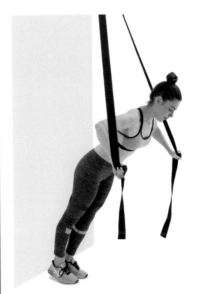

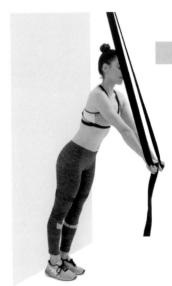

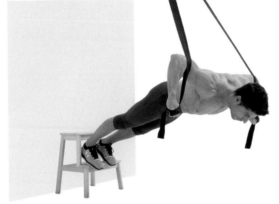

STARTING POSITION

Harder variation

The principal exercise provides maximum intensity at its lowest phase, namely, when the body is parallel to the ground. Nonetheless, placing your feet on an elevated spot will make it possible for you to go further than horizontal, involve more of your deltoid muscles, and work at angles and resistance levels that are almost impossible. This is only appropriate for very experienced exercisers and with very tough supports.

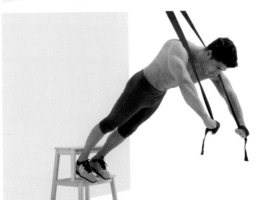

FINAL POSITION

03 Deep Push-Ups With Supports

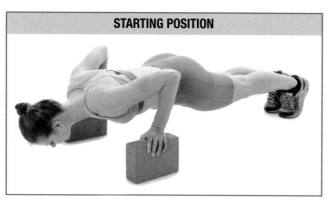

STARTING POSITION

The variation with supports makes it possible to move the chest to a point that is lower than the hand supports. The movement is longer and the worked muscles start from a more stretched position in relation to that of a normal push-up, which increases the intensity and difficulty of the exercise.

Execution

Use a pair of supports for your hands; these can be thick books, stools or anything else which enables you to keep your body above the level of the ground.

Put yourself in push-up position with your toes pressed into the ground, your trunk and lower extremities aligned, and the palms of your hands on the supports.

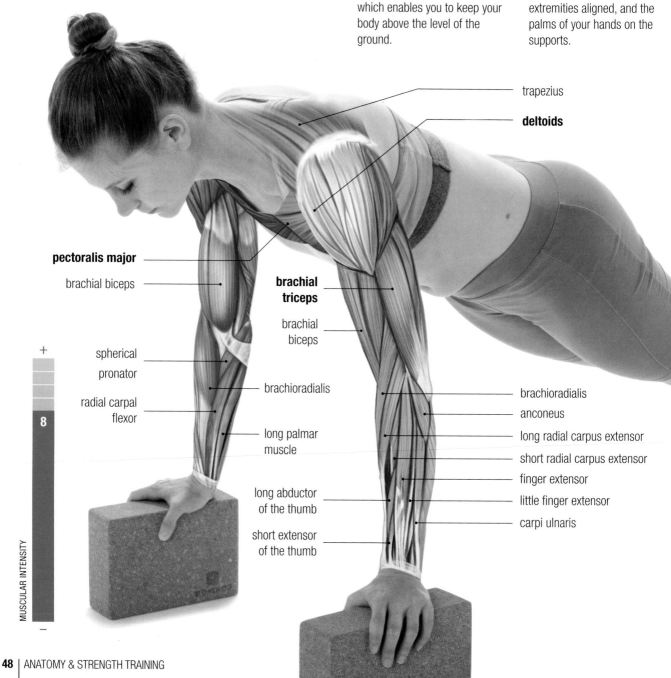

trapezius

deltoids

pectoralis major

brachial biceps

brachial triceps

brachial biceps

spherical pronator

radial carpal flexor

brachioradialis

brachioradialis

anconeus

long radial carpus extensor

short radial carpus extensor

finger extensor

little finger extensor

carpi ulnaris

long palmar muscle

long abductor of the thumb

short extensor of the thumb

+

8

−

MUSCULAR INTENSITY

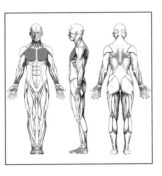

Technical considerations

- Keep your trunk and lower extremities aligned.

- Check to be sure that your supporting items are stable.

- Lower your chest below the level of your hands.

- Go as far as possible.

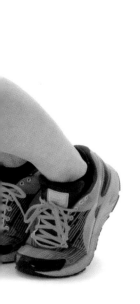

▬ Easier variation

In order to support your hands, you can begin with two higher supports, for example, the backs of chairs. This will position you more perpendicularly in relation to the ground and as the inclination is reduced, the difficulty of the exercise is also reduced. This is a good alternative if the previous suggestion is too complicated for you to execute.

STARTING POSITION

FINAL POSITION

STARTING POSITION

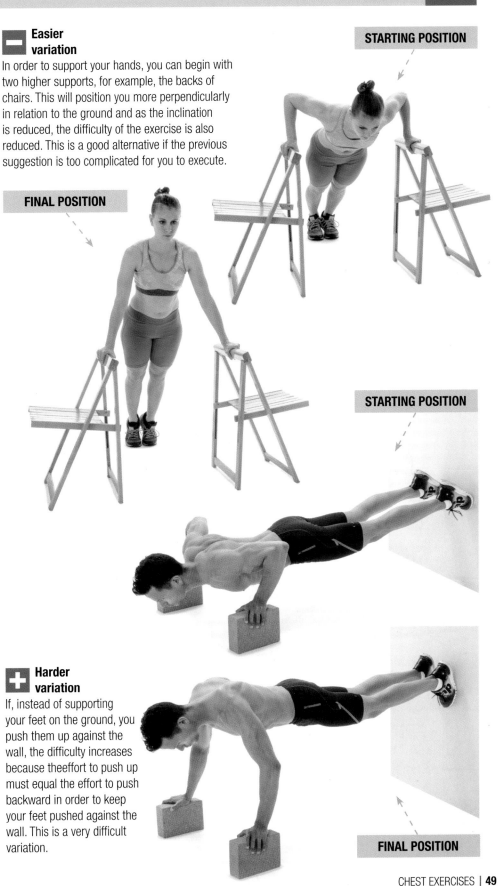

✚ Harder variation

If, instead of supporting your feet on the ground, you push them up against the wall, the difficulty increases because theeffort to push up must equal the effort to push backward in order to keep your feet pushed against the wall. This is a very difficult variation.

FINAL POSITION

04 Lateral Push-Ups

This is one of the numerous variations of traditional push-ups. This is a classic exercise that has been modified and reinvented many times. Here, the lateral push-ups have a greater level of difficulty, and doing them correctly involves a challenge even for the most experienced exercisers.

Execution

Put yourself in push-up position, but do not flex your elbows to the same extent, nor completely lower yourself to the ground. Instead of this, tilt upward. One of your elbows will flex a lot and the opposite only a little. Thus, the torso will be over one hand and away from the other. Go back up and then back down, moving your body toward the opposite side. You can return to the starting point each time, or just move from side to side.

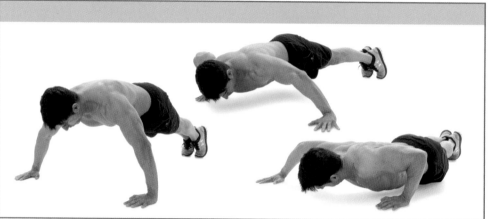

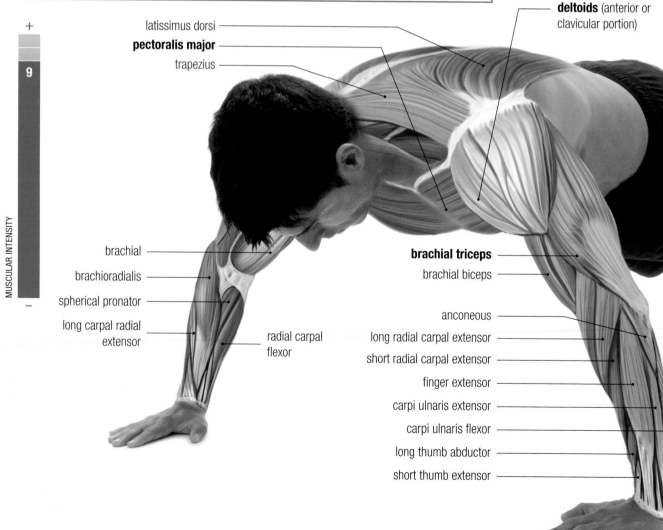

MUSCULAR INTENSITY

+

9

−

latissimus dorsi

pectoralis major

trapezius

deltoids (anterior or clavicular portion)

brachial

brachioradialis

spherical pronator

long carpal radial extensor

radial carpal flexor

brachial triceps

brachial biceps

anconeous

long radial carpal extensor

short radial carpal extensor

finger extensor

carpi ulnaris extensor

carpi ulnaris flexor

long thumb abductor

short thumb extensor

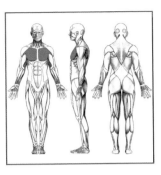

Technical considerations

■ The separation between your hands should be greater than the separation used in classic push-ups.

■ Your trunk and lower extremities must be in perfect alignment.

■ You can modify the exercise by focusing more on the ascent and descent of your chest or on its lateral movement.

➖ Easier variation

Lie with your back on the seat of a chair and hold on to the back of the chair with one hand. Hold a water jug with the other hand as you do this.

Your elbow will be extended, and the water jug will be at one side of your body. Keeping your elbow slightly, but continuously flexed, lift the water jug until it is above your chest. You can do the same exercise as flexing and extending the elbow like in a chest press.

STARTING POSITION

FINAL POSITION

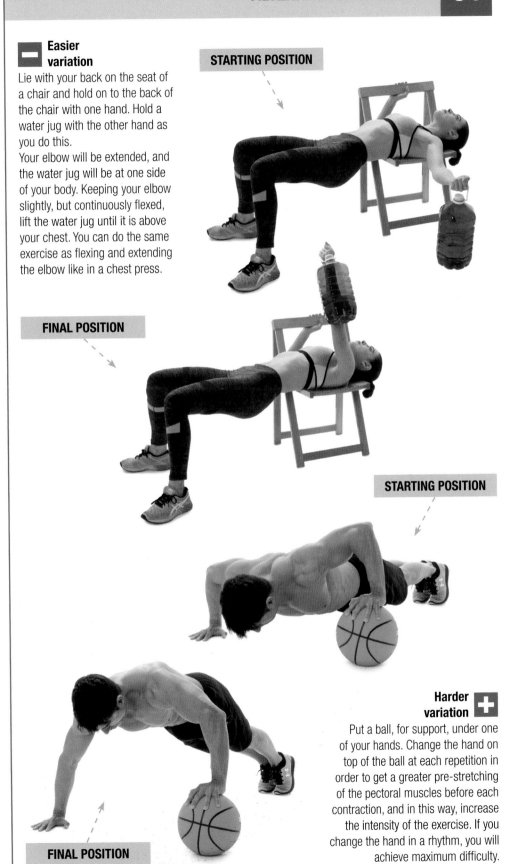

STARTING POSITION

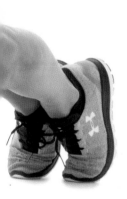

FINAL POSITION

➕ Harder variation

Put a ball, for support, under one of your hands. Change the hand on top of the ball at each repetition in order to get a greater pre-stretching of the pectoral muscles before each contraction, and in this way, increase the intensity of the exercise. If you change the hand in a rhythm, you will achieve maximum difficulty.

05 Sliding Push-Ups With Towels

Push-ups, whether with machines, dumbbells, or pulleys, are muscle movements for the pectoral muscles which generally use press movements. In this case, with the assumption of not having any specific equipment, one of the customary options is to work on the ground and use body weight. A pair of towels can facilitate the sliding of the hands.

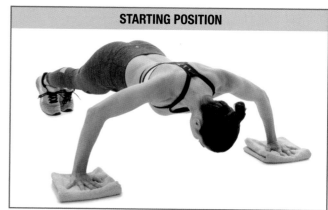

STARTING POSITION

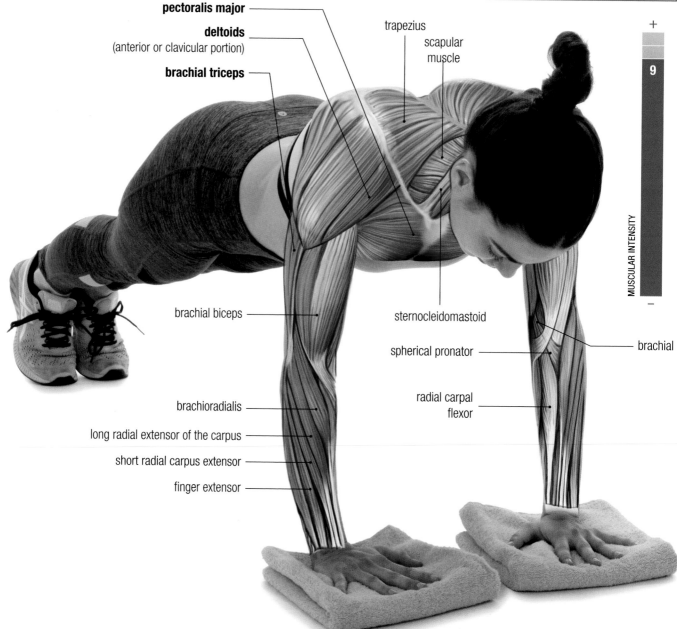

pectoralis major

deltoids
(anterior or clavicular portion)

brachial triceps

trapezius

scapular muscle

brachial biceps

sternocleidomastoid

spherical pronator

brachial

brachioradialis

radial carpal flexor

long radial extensor of the carpus

short radial carpus extensor

finger extensor

MUSCULAR INTENSITY

+

9

−

ALTERNATIVE EXERCISES | 05

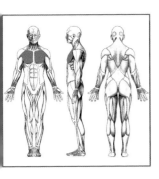

Execution

Put yourself in the push-up position, supporting each hand on a small towel or other item which will make it possible for you to slide along the floor. Separate your hands so that your chest nears the ground. Stop at the lowest point and try to move your hands back together in order to return them to the starting position. This is something that not everyone will be able to do.

Technical considerations

- Keep your trunk and lower extremities aligned.

- Gently and progressively flex your elbows while you lower your body and extend them again as you come back up.

- As your level advances, you will have to separate your hands more in order to get the greatest benefit from the exercise.

— Easier variation

The same exercise can be done using the wall with a much smaller inclination of the body, which will involve less difficulty. This changes the exercise from a very intense floor exercise to a very easy wall exercise, which is ideal if you are a beginner.

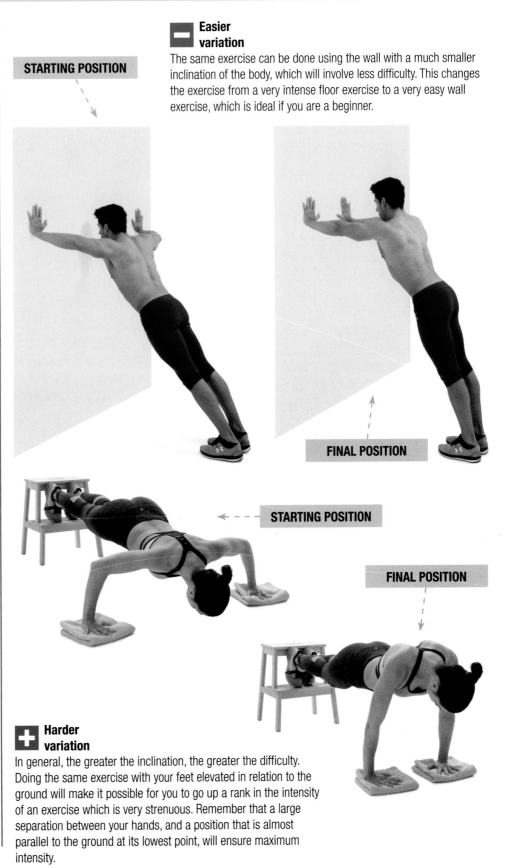

STARTING POSITION

FINAL POSITION

STARTING POSITION

FINAL POSITION

+ Harder variation

In general, the greater the inclination, the greater the difficulty. Doing the same exercise with your feet elevated in relation to the ground will make it possible for you to go up a rank in the intensity of an exercise which is very strenuous. Remember that a large separation between your hands, and a position that is almost parallel to the ground at its lowest point, will ensure maximum intensity.

06 Jump Push-Ups

A push-up movement can be done by adding modifications such as inclination, position and separation of the hands, distance moved or, as in this exercise, by providing additional speed and converting it into an explosive movement such as a pitch or a jump. Don't forget to do a thorough warm-up before performing explosive movements.

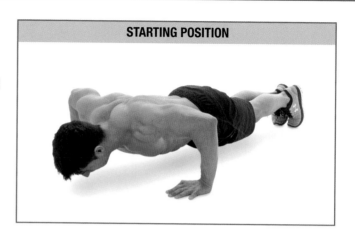

STARTING POSITION

+

8

MUSCULAR INTENSITY

−

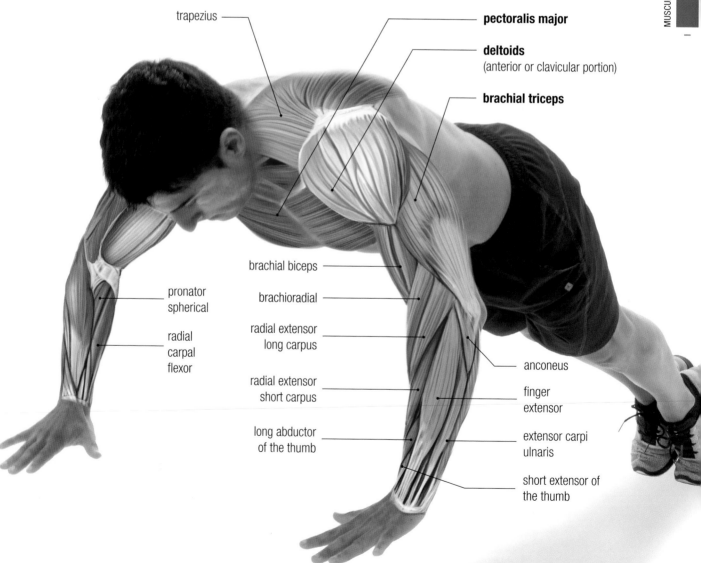

trapezius

pectoralis major

deltoids
(anterior or clavicular portion)

brachial triceps

brachial biceps

brachioradial

pronator spherical

radial extensor long carpus

radial carpal flexor

anconeus

radial extensor short carpus

finger extensor

long abductor of the thumb

extensor carpi ulnaris

short extensor of the thumb

ALTERNATIVE EXERCISES 06

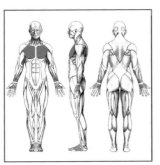

Execution

Beginning in the push-up position, lower the chest until you reach the lowest point of the movement.

From there, push yourself upward with strength and speed, generating enough power so that the movement does not stop when you extend your elbows, but rather becomes longer with both hands lifting off from the floor, and executing a small jump.

Technical considerations

- Do a thorough warm-up before doing power exercises.

- When your hands reconnect with the floor, flex your elbows to soften your fall and prevent damage to your elbows and wrists.

- Keep your trunk and lower extremities aligned at all times.

Easier variation

Decreasing the inclination of the body will decrease the difficulty of the exercise. For beginning athletes, doing the exercise against the wall is a good option. At the lowest point of the exercise, the body will be tilted forward, and when you push off, you should be almost perpendicular to the floor.

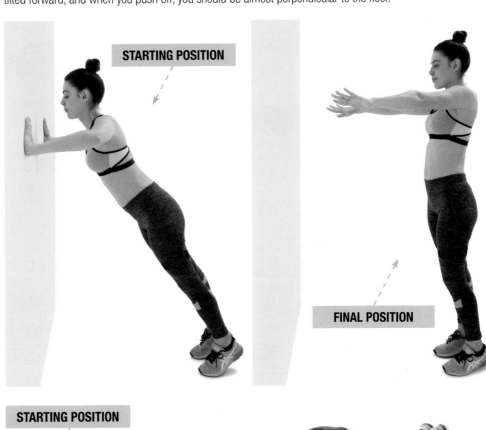

STARTING POSITION

FINAL POSITION

STARTING POSITION

FINAL POSITION

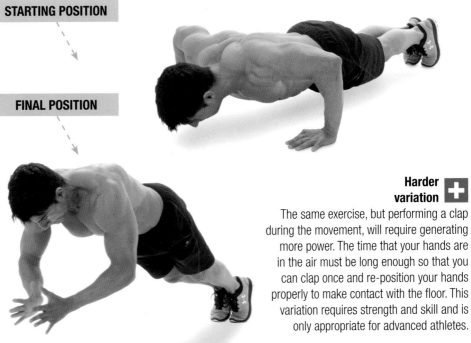

Harder variation

The same exercise, but performing a clap during the movement, will require generating more power. The time that your hands are in the air must be long enough so that you can clap once and re-position your hands properly to make contact with the floor. This variation requires strength and skill and is only appropriate for advanced athletes.

07 Push-Ups With Retracted Hands

This is one of the multiple variations of classic push-ups. This time, the difficulty is increased by retracting the hands, which moves the work toward the lower fibers of the pectoralis major and the anterior deltoids.

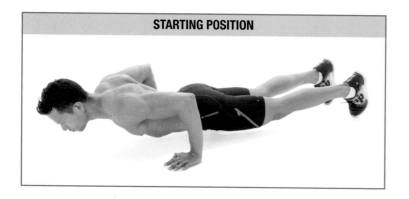

STARTING POSITION

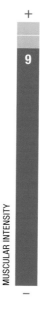

+

9

−

MUSCULAR INTENSITY

Execution
Lie facedown with the palms of your hands on the floor. Do not place your hands next to your chest, but rather at a point that is further back, beside your abdomen. Push upward until your elbows are almost completely extended.

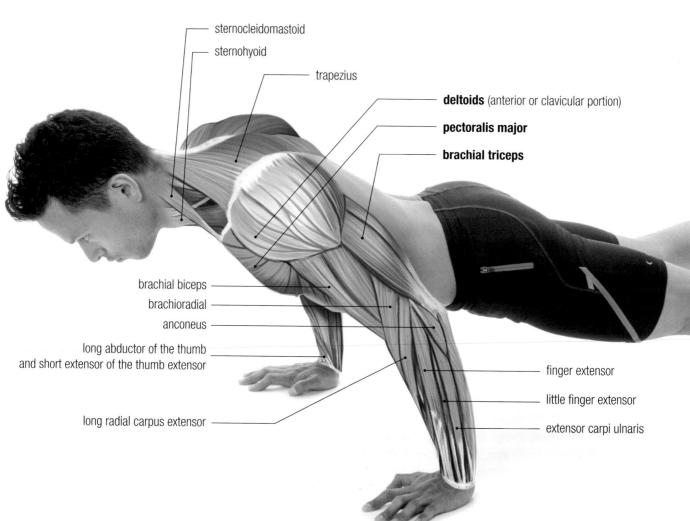

sternocleidomastoid

sternohyoid

trapezius

deltoids (anterior or clavicular portion)

pectoralis major

brachial triceps

brachial biceps

brachioradial

anconeus

long abductor of the thumb and short extensor of the thumb extensor

long radial carpus extensor

finger extensor

little finger extensor

extensor carpi ulnaris

ALTERNATIVE EXERCISES 07

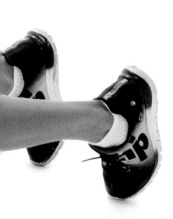

Technical considerations

■ Keep your trunk and lower extremities aligned.

■ First try the exercise with only a slight retraction of the hands and continue to increase this retraction as your ability to execute the exercise increases.

■ If you feel pain in your wrists, turn the hand support so that your fingers face outward.

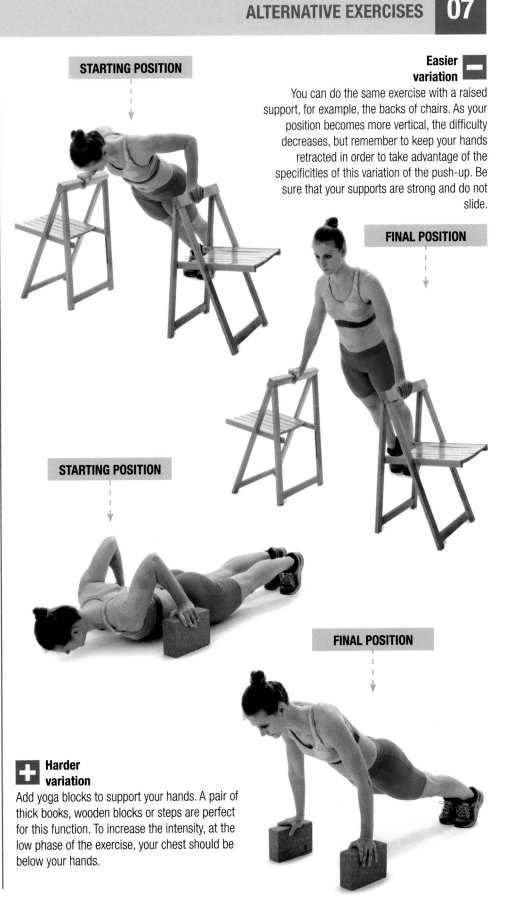

STARTING POSITION

Easier variation

You can do the same exercise with a raised support, for example, the backs of chairs. As your position becomes more vertical, the difficulty decreases, but remember to keep your hands retracted in order to take advantage of the specificities of this variation of the push-up. Be sure that your supports are strong and do not slide.

FINAL POSITION

STARTING POSITION

FINAL POSITION

➕ Harder variation

Add yoga blocks to support your hands. A pair of thick books, wooden blocks or steps are perfect for this function. To increase the intensity, at the low phase of the exercise, your chest should be below your hands.

08 | Suspension Row

STARTING POSITION

Rows and pull-ups are classic muscle movements for the back and are customarily done by athletes of all levels at fitness centers. Not having equipment to do these exercises is not an obstacle to reaping the benefits of their effectiveness, since there are many variations that require little more than our own body weight.

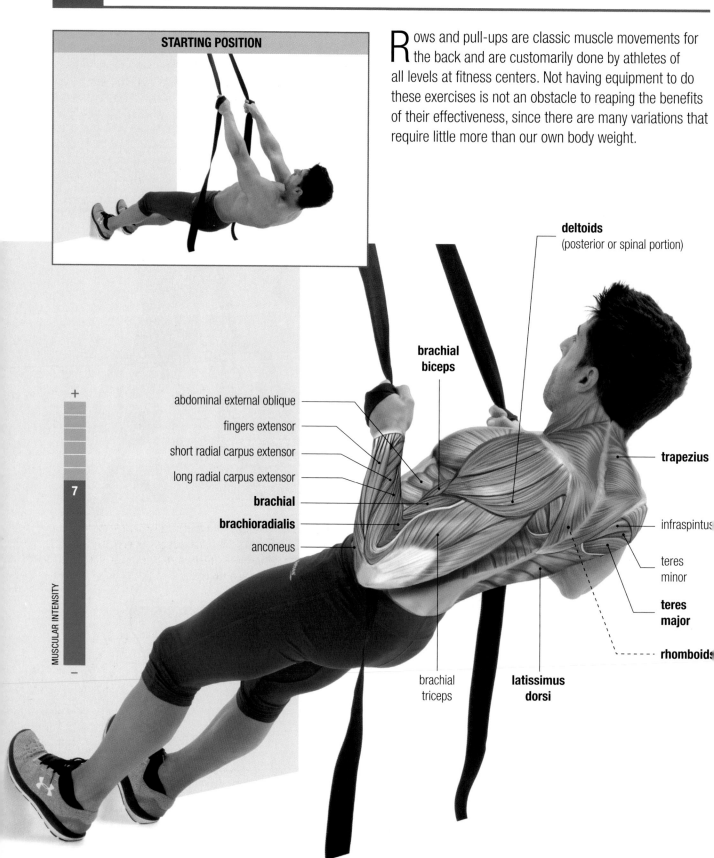

MUSCULAR INTENSITY

+

7

−

abdominal external oblique

fingers extensor

short radial carpus extensor

long radial carpus extensor

brachial

brachioradialis

anconeus

brachial biceps

brachial triceps

latissimus dorsi

deltoids
(posterior or spinal portion)

trapezius

infraspintus

teres minor

teres major

rhomboids

ALTERNATIVE EXERCISES 08

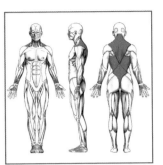

Execution

Put a nylon belt, or a suspension training device if you have one, over an elevated support. Hold each end of the belt with one hand, and lean back until you are suspended and your elbows are extended. Your feet can be against the wall or, if this is not possible, on the ground. Bend your elbows so that your torso moves up.

Technical considerations

■ Try to keep your chest out, contract your back and push your shoulders back at the highest point of the movement.

■ Keep your thighs and trunk aligned.

■ Consider increasing the inclination if the difficulty is insufficient.

■ If you tend to move laterally, separate your feet to improve your stability.

▬ Easier variation

Reducing the inclination of the body until you are almost standing at the highest point of the movement is a variation of the principal exercise, which makes its execution easier, especially for beginning athletes. Starting there, continue to release the belt until you have reached a suitable inclination.

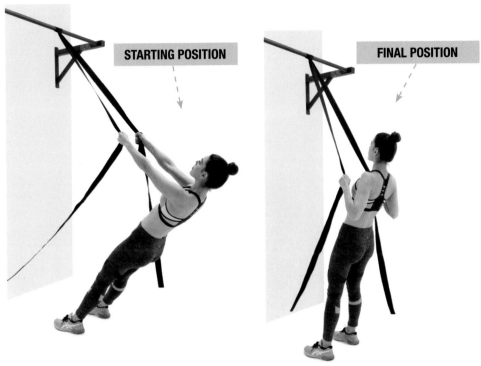

STARTING POSITION

FINAL POSITION

➕ Harder variation

Putting your feet on an elevated surface will increase the difficulty of the principal exercise. You will be able to achieve a position parallel to the floor at the lowest point of the exercise, or even have your shoulders lower than your feet if you are a very experienced athlete. Remember that your feet must be well supported so that they do not fall and so that you do not run any risk.

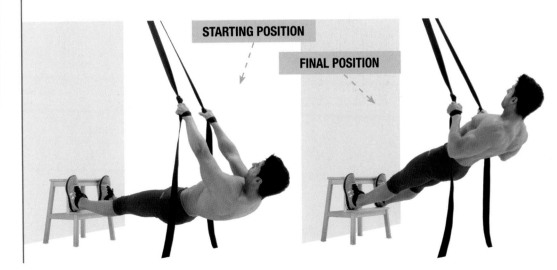

STARTING POSITION

FINAL POSITION

09 Inverted Row With Bar

This variation of the row with a traditional bar makes it possible for you to substitute your body weight for the weight provided by a bar and the disks. A heavy table or other fixed items in parks or urban spaces, such as a railing, provide ideal support for you to hang from.

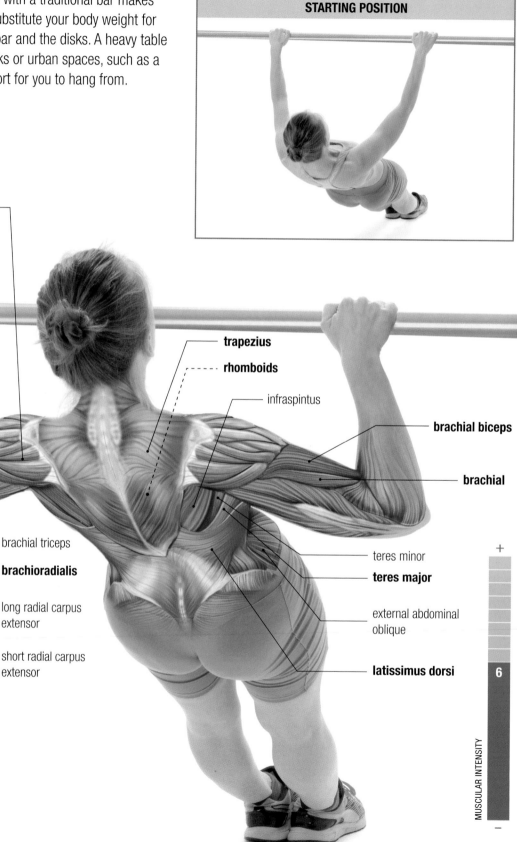

STARTING POSITION

deltoids
(posterior or spinal portion)

trapezius

rhomboids

infraspintus

brachial biceps

brachial

brachial triceps

brachioradialis

long radial carpus extensor

short radial carpus extensor

teres minor

teres major

external abdominal oblique

latissimus dorsi

MUSCULAR INTENSITY

+

6

−

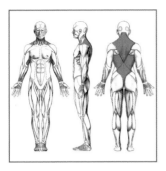

Execution

Stand under a support and grip it firmly with both hands, with your hands placed outside of your shoulders. Align your legs and trunk so that you are hanging from the support with your elbows extended, keeping your heels in contact with the ground. Pull on the bar and try to raise your chest as close to it as possible, overcoming your own weight.

Technical considerations

- Keep your trunk and lower extremities aligned.

- Concentrate your efforts in your back muscles and avoid doing the work with your arms.

- Move your chest as close to the bar as you can.

Easier variation

In order to reduce intensity, or during the first weeks of training, you can execute this type of rowing, standing up and using a pair of water bottles, which can be filled higher in order to progressively increase the resistance. Remember to keep your knees slightly flexed and your trunk inclined. However, your back should remain straight in order to avoid injuries.

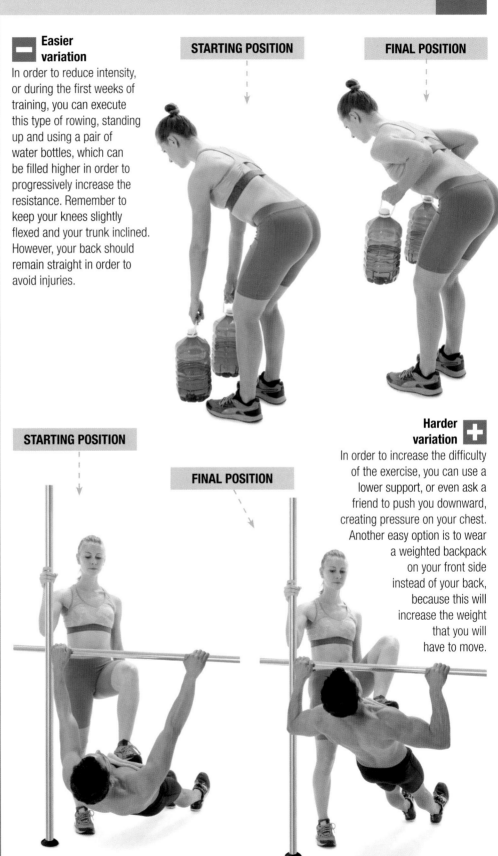

STARTING POSITION

FINAL POSITION

STARTING POSITION

FINAL POSITION

Harder variation

In order to increase the difficulty of the exercise, you can use a lower support, or even ask a friend to push you downward, creating pressure on your chest. Another easy option is to wear a weighted backpack on your front side instead of your back, because this will increase the weight that you will have to move.

10 Chin-Ups With Weight

Chin-ups are a customary exercise for strengthening the latissimus dorsi. A strong tree branch, a girder or any other solid construction from which you can hang can be used for this exercise. Who has never been tempted to do a chin up when seeing a solid city construction that offers itself for just that purpose?

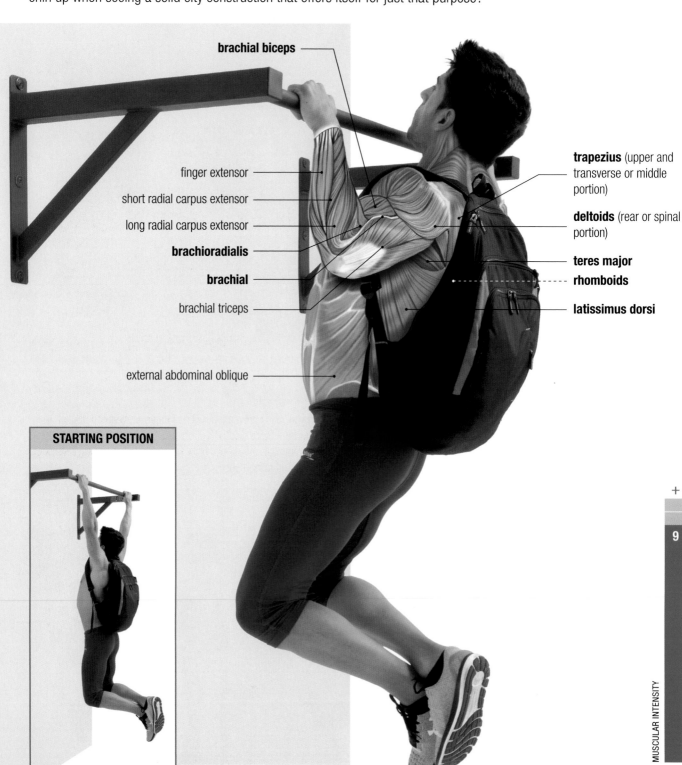

brachial biceps

finger extensor

short radial carpus extensor

long radial carpus extensor

brachioradialis

brachial

brachial triceps

external abdominal oblique

trapezius (upper and transverse or middle portion)

deltoids (rear or spinal portion)

teres major

rhomboids

latissimus dorsi

STARTING POSITION

MUSCULAR INTENSITY

+

9

−

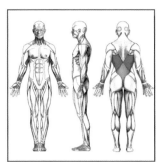

Execution

Hang from a solid construction by both hands so that your hands are separated and your elbows are extended. In order to increase the difficulty, we suggest that you add a weight to an exercise that is already hard for you. Fill a backpack with books or other items that add weight, and make the execution of the exercise more difficult by placing the backpack on your back. Once you are hanging from the bar, try to move up using shoulder adduction and flexing your elbows until your chin is over the height of the bar.

Technical considerations

■ The separation between your hands should be greater than that between your shoulders.

■ Try to focus the effort on your back muscles and lighten the work for your elbow flexors.

■ Try to reach the bar with your chin.

▬ Easier variation

If you eliminate the weight, this same exercise will be less difficult. This does not mean that it will become a basic for beginners, since chin ups always involve a medium to high level of difficulty. If you are a beginner, a chin-up may be too difficult for you.

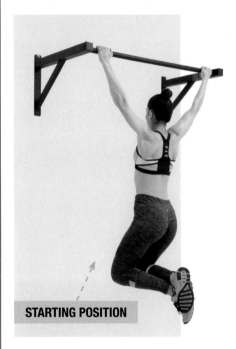

STARTING POSITION

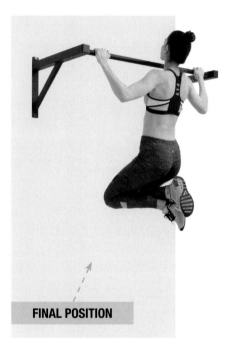

FINAL POSITION

✚ Harder variation

Execute the chin-up on one side so that as your body moves up, it is no longer between hands but instead moving toward one of them. Starting from there, you will be able to lower yourself again and move back up toward the other side, or you can even move your body from side to side, always staying in the highest zone, which is an extremely difficult movement.

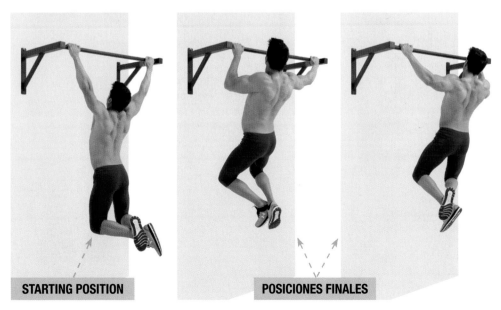

STARTING POSITION

POSICIONES FINALES

11 Pull-Ups With Closed, Reverse Grip

Climbing movements develop the latissimus dorsi efficiently, and for this reason, pull-ups are very popular with bodybuilding athletes. There are a multitude of variations with almost inexhaustible possibilities for working the back. From among these, the variation with closed, reverse group is probably one of the most effective.

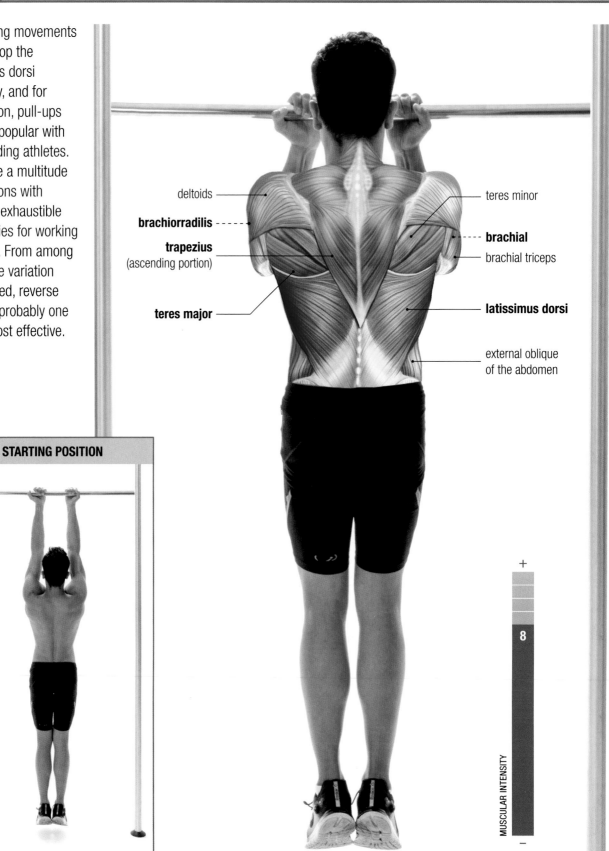

deltoids

brachiorradilis

trapezius
(ascending portion)

teres major

teres minor

brachial

brachial triceps

latissimus dorsi

external oblique
of the abdomen

STARTING POSITION

MUSCULAR INTENSITY

+

8

−

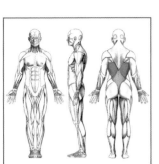

Execution

Use a vertical support that resists traction like those in public parks or open-air training areas. Hold the bar with both hands in the supine position. Pull up to lift your own weight and try to move your chin level with or above the height of the bar.

Technical considerations

- Your feet should not be touching the ground.

- If the support is not high enough, you should bend your knees.

- Try to concentrate the effort in your latissimus dorsi and minimize the involvement of the brachial biceps.

- Complete one repetition so that in the lower phase of the exercise, your elbows are extended.

STARTING POSITION

Easier variation —

Lie down on a bench and hold the one end of a belt or cord in each hand. Your partner will hold the cord by its center and will pull and release the cord always providing resistance, while you perform the opposite action.

FINAL POSITION

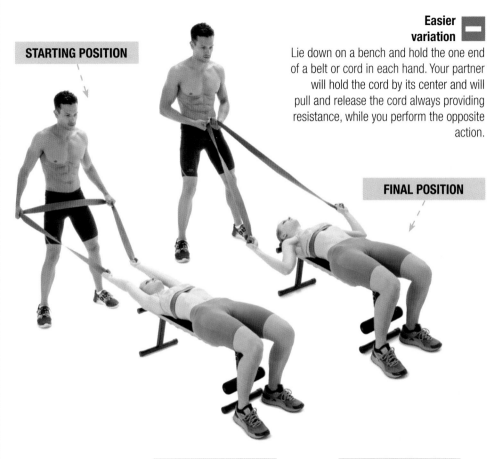

Harder variation +

One-arm pull-ups with reverse grip are a challenge, even for advanced athletes. Hang by one hand while you hold your wrist with the other hand and try to pull yourself up until your chin reaches the height of the bar. Completing only 5 or 6 repetitions will be a real challenge.

STARTING POSITION

FINAL POSITION

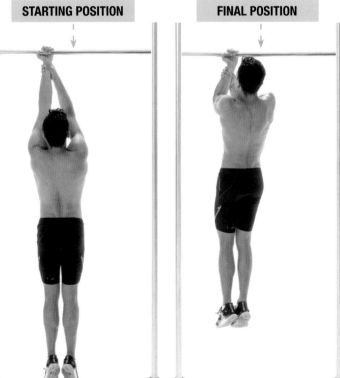

12 | **Commando Pull-Ups**

The commando pull-up is one of the least seen variations in gyms frequented by bodybuilders. However, it is very popular with athletes who practice calisthenics and have great potential for developing the strength and volume of the musculature of the back.

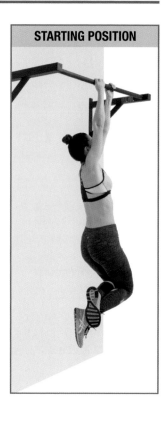

STARTING POSITION

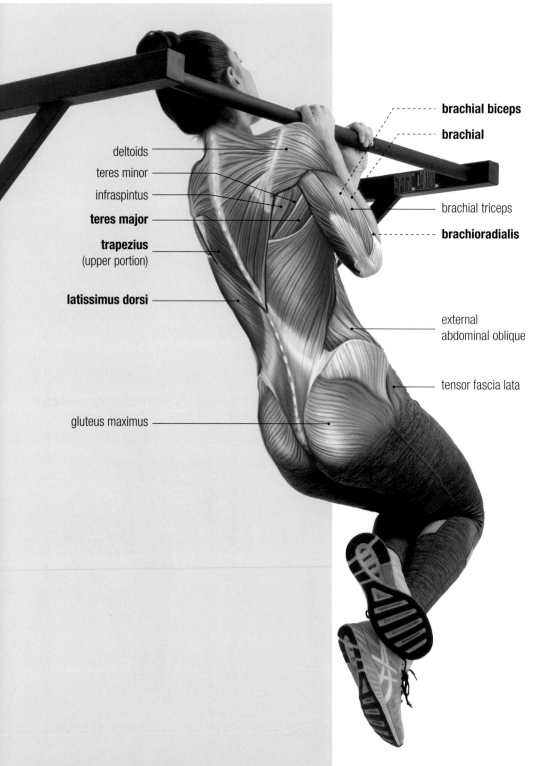

deltoids

teres minor

infraspintus

teres major

trapezius
(upper portion)

latissimus dorsi

gluteus maximus

brachial biceps

brachial

brachial triceps

brachioradialis

external
abdominal oblique

tensor fascia lata

MUSCULAR INTENSITY

+

8

−

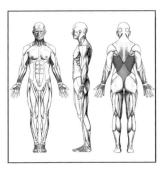

Execution

Hold on to a horizontal, elevated and fixed support. Place your hands in a neutral position, one in front of the other so that you are hanging with your elbows extended.

Then, pull up on the bar while moving your head to one side of it until your shoulder touches it. Let yourself back down, and then repeat the exercise, moving your head to the opposite side of the bar.

Technical considerations

- Concentrate all of the effort in your back muscles and minimize the work of the elbow flexing muscles.

- Complete the repetitions placing your head on one side or alternatively the other side of the bar.

- Try to get your shoulder as close to the bar as possible.

✚ Easier variation

In this first higher intensity alternative, you will have to use a grip with a greater separation between your hands and then move your chest to the bar so that your body moves toward a horizontal position, as it rises. The more parallel to the bar you are in the final phase of the exercise, the greater the effort required.

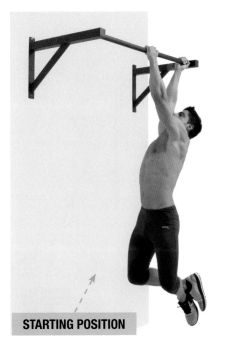

STARTING POSITION

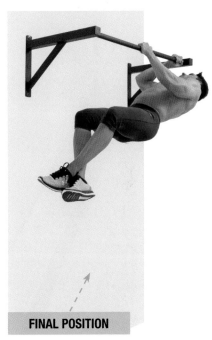

FINAL POSITION

✚ Harder variation

This variation is a little less extreme than the previous one so we suggest doing it with an added weight. A backpack is a good option since it can be filled to a greater or lesser degree, but holding a weight with your legs or feet is also a good alternative.

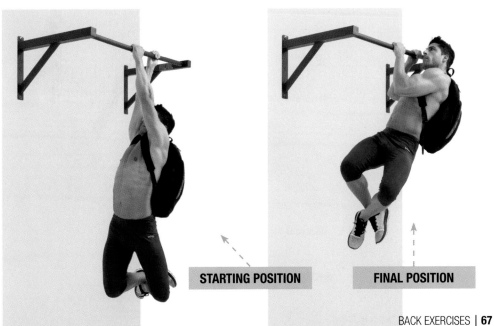

STARTING POSITION

FINAL POSITION

13 Row With Support and Weights

Any lack of specialized equipment can almost always be remediated with some simple items and a bit of imagination. Here, we substitute the classic rowing machine or the pulley rower with a nylon belt, a weight and a support to pass the belt over; the obtained result is equivalent to that achieved with the traditional equipment.

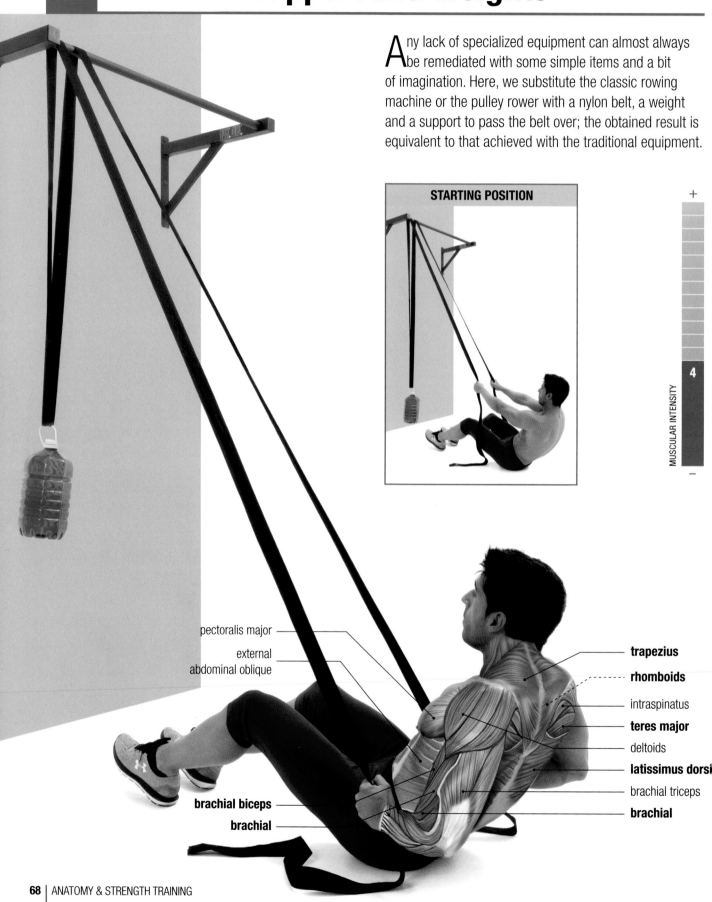

STARTING POSITION

MUSCULAR INTENSITY

+

4

−

pectoralis major

external abdominal oblique

trapezius

rhomboids

intraspinatus

teres major

deltoids

latissimus dorsi

brachial triceps

brachial biceps

brachial

brachial

ALTERNATIVE EXERCISES **13**

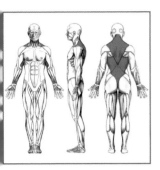

Execution

Pass the belt through the handle of a water jug and then over an elevated support. Sit down, hold each one of the ends of the belt with one hand and lean back slightly so that your elbows are extended and the weight is hanging. Pull back with both hands, sliding the belt and moving the weight up in a rowing movement.

Technical considerations

- The smoother the support, the less friction there will be on the belt and the more similar the resistance, provided by the weight in going up and down.

- Try to focus the effort on your back muscles and lighten the work for your brachial biceps.

▬ Easier variation

Pass the belt over the support and pull one end with each hand until it is tight. Pull with one arm and flex the elbow in a rowing movement, while the opposite arm, which is moving forward extends with resistance. Then, execute the reverse movement so that each side works against the resistance of the opposite side.

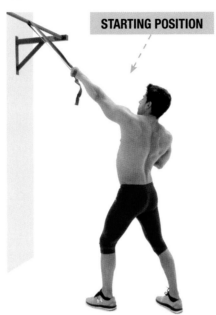

STARTING POSITION

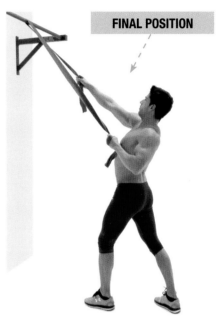

FINAL POSITION

✚ Harder variation

This variation consists of performing the principal exercise on one side, which requires you to hold both ends of the belt in the same hand. Do the exercise this way if the weights you have are not heavy enough to do the exercise bilaterally.

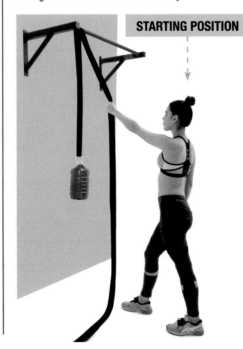

STARTING POSITION

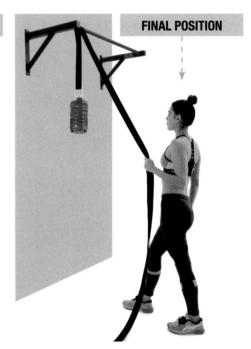

FINAL POSITION

14 Suspension Pull-Over

The classic pull-over movement can be modified to provide greater effectiveness without the need for bars, dumbbells or pulleys. Body weight, a cord and an anchoring point make it possible to reap the benefits of the pullover with minimum equipment.

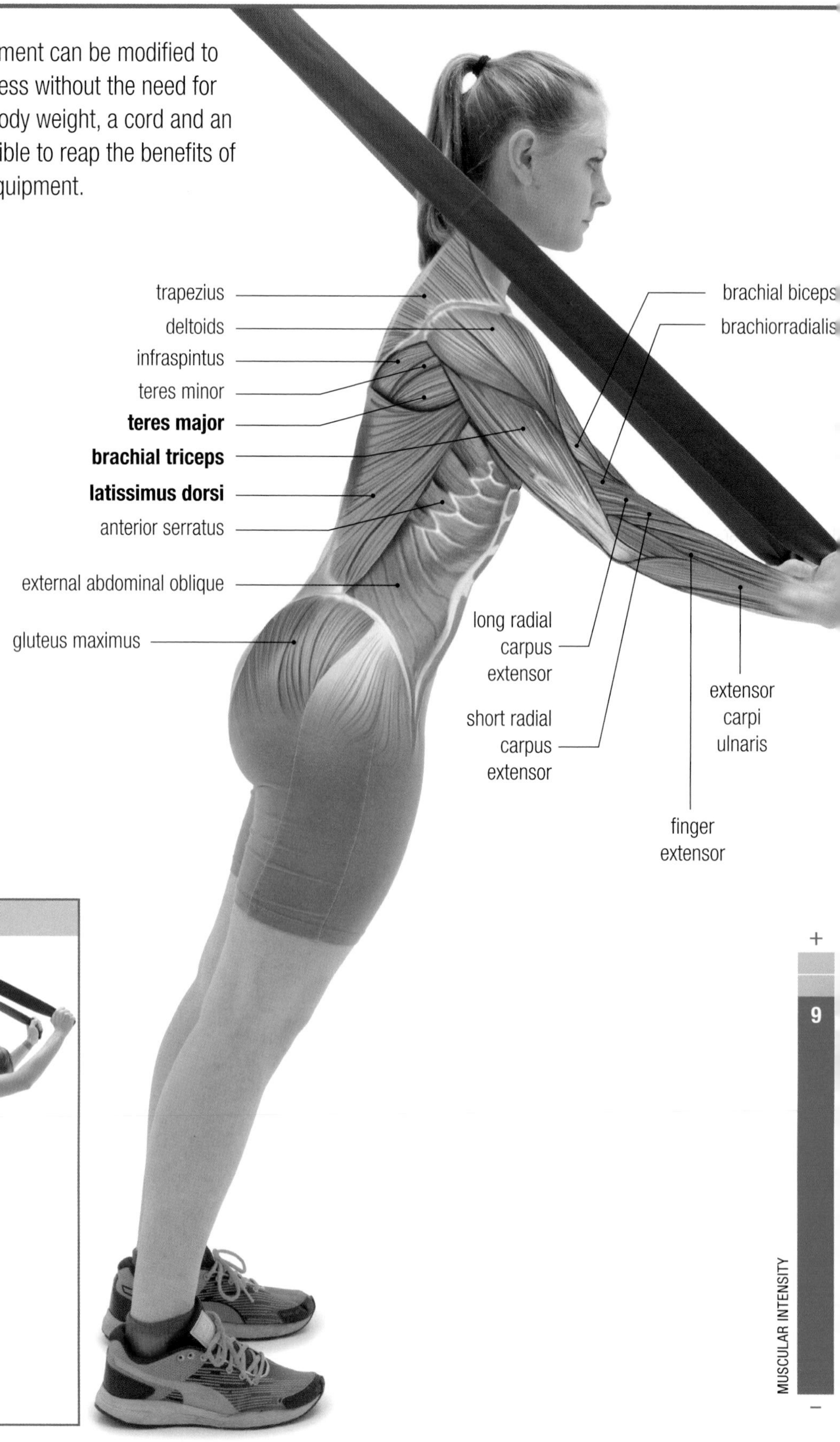

trapezius

deltoids

infraspintus

teres minor

teres major

brachial triceps

latissimus dorsi

anterior serratus

external abdominal oblique

gluteus maximus

brachial biceps

brachiorradialis

long radial carpus extensor

short radial carpus extensor

extensor carpi ulnaris

finger extensor

STARTING POSITION

+

9

MUSCULAR INTENSITY

−

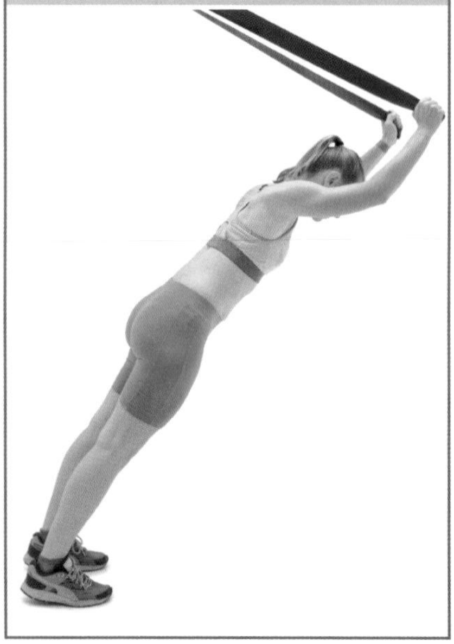

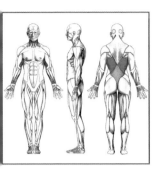

Execution

Pass a cord or a nylon belt through an elevated anchoring point such as a strong tree branch or a beam. Hold both ends of the belt at the same time as you extend your shoulders and elbows, and lean forward. You should be standing on your toes and hanging from the cords. Lift your hands toward the front until they are in front of your chest and you are lifting your own weight and becoming more perpendicular in relation to the floor.

Technical considerations

- Your lower extremities and trunk must remain aligned through the entire exercise.

- Your elbows will be almost completely extended from the beginning to the end of the exercise.

- Separate your feet so that you will be sufficiently balanced throughout the exercise.

▬ Easier variation

Support your back on a bench or seat, and try to execute the classic pull-over using one or two water jugs which can be full or empty, depending on the resistance required. It will be sufficient to support your upper back to execute this low difficulty variation.

STARTING POSITION

FINAL POSITION

✚ Harder variation

To increase the difficulty of the suspended pull-over, it is necessary to increase your inclination. The more inclined you are in the starting position, the harder the exercise will be, up to the point that you begin almost parallel to the floor, which is the position of maximum effort, even for the most advanced athletes.

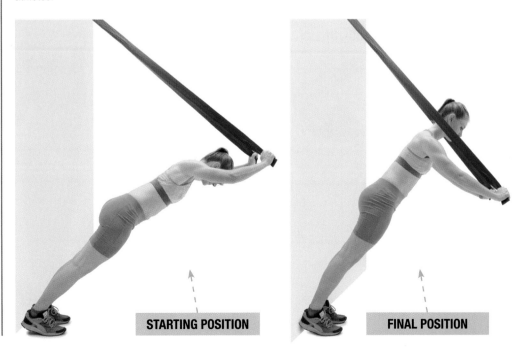

STARTING POSITION   **FINAL POSITION**

15 Shrugs

Shrugs are the basic bodybuilding movement for developing the upper trapezius, its descending fibers. Nonetheless, many of the movements used to train the deltoids, such as rowing to the forehead, lateral raises or shoulder presses, will also develop this portion of the trapezius.

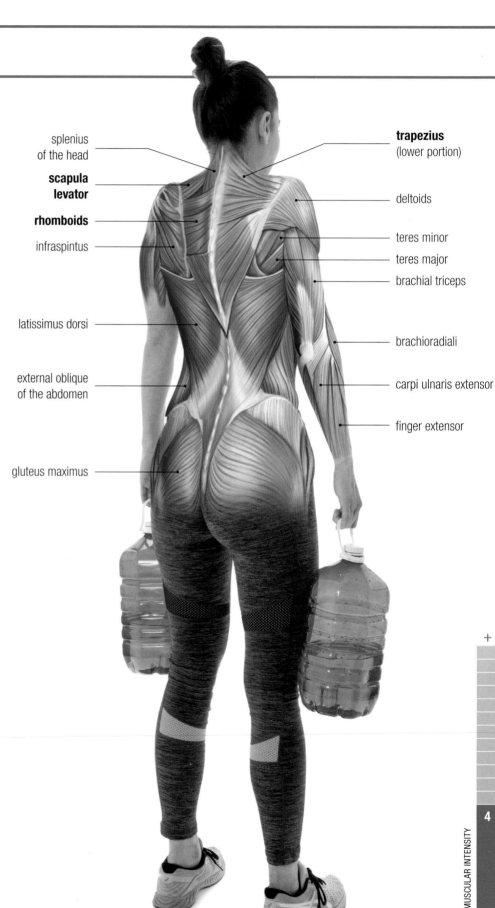

splenius of the head

scapula levator

rhomboids

infraspintus

latissimus dorsi

external oblique of the abdomen

gluteus maximus

trapezius (lower portion)

deltoids

teres minor

teres major

brachial triceps

brachioradiali

carpi ulnaris extensor

finger extensor

STARTING POSITION

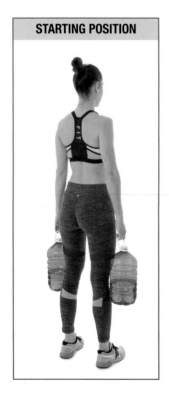

MUSCULAR INTENSITY

4

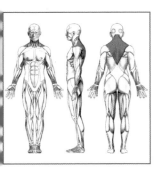

Execution

Starting from a standing position, hold a weight with each hand so that the weights are hanging at your sides. Water jugs, used as weights, make it possible to regulate the weight and, more importantly be certain that the weights are the same on both sides.

Keep your elbows extended and your shoulders relaxed. From this point, raise your shoulders without moving your elbows.

Technical considerations

- Do not move your arms backward while raising your shoulders.

- Do not lock your knees in extended position but rather, flex them slightly, especially when you are lifting a heavy weight.

- Keep your back straight.

➖ Easier variation

In this variation, a partner supports their hands over yours and regulates the resistance while doing the movement. If you are training alone, you can do the same exercise holding onto the end of a table and pulling it up and down; in this way, you will be able to work with reduced resistance.

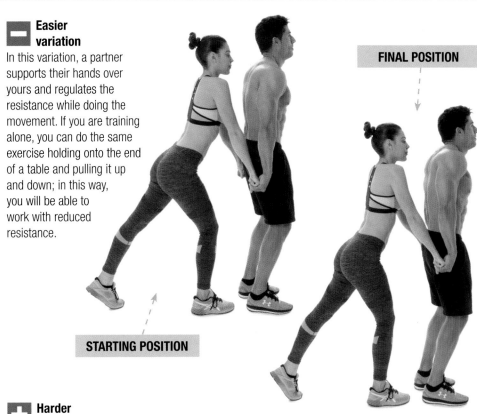

FINAL POSITION

STARTING POSITION

➕ Harder variation

The starting point is the same as for the principal exercise, but instead of the ascending-descending rear movement, it is a counterclockwise movement, going from bottom to front to top to back, and back to the beginning. Although the intensity is not greatly increased, there are a greater number of muscles involved.

SEQUENCE

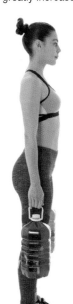
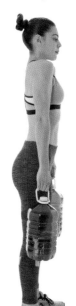
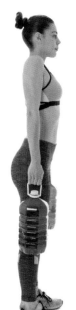
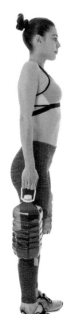
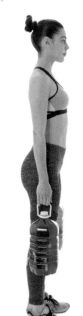

16 | Double Arch

The double arch works the spinal erector muscles. These muscles are completely forgotten in the major bodybuilding disciplines since they are deep and inconspicuous, but they have an essential role to play in correct posture and balance of the spine.

STARTING POSITION

Execution
Lie facedown, with your legs and arms extended. From this position, try to arch your body so that your arms and legs are raised, separating from the floor with your spine maximally extended. Despite how it may appear, a good final position will be difficult to achieve and even more difficult to maintain.

+

9

MUSCULAR INTENSITY

−

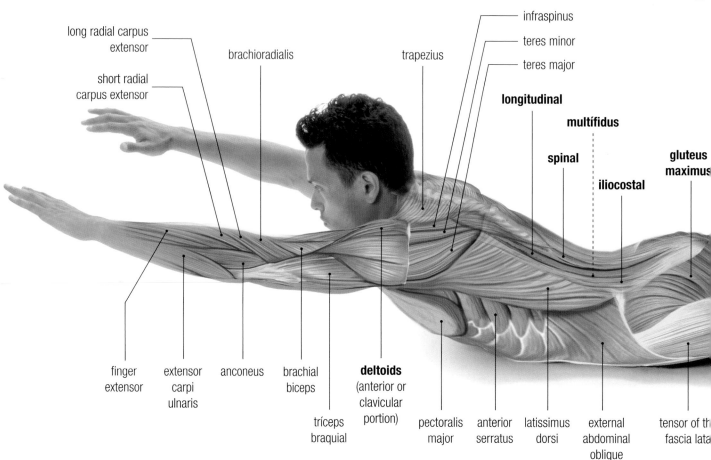

long radial carpus extensor

short radial carpus extensor

brachioradialis

trapezius

infraspinus

teres minor

teres major

longitudinal

multífidus

spinal

iliocostal

gluteus maximus

finger extensor

extensor carpi ulnaris

anconeus

brachial biceps

tríceps braquial

deltoids (anterior or clavicular portion)

pectoralis major

anterior serratus

latissimus dorsi

external abdominal oblique

tensor of the fascia lata

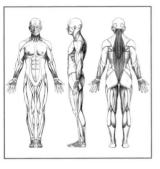

Technical considerations

■ At the moment of maximum contraction, only your abdomen should be supported.

■ Be sure that your thighs and chest are separated from the floor when you reach the final position.

■ A good option is to complete a smaller number of repetitions, but hold the final position for several seconds.

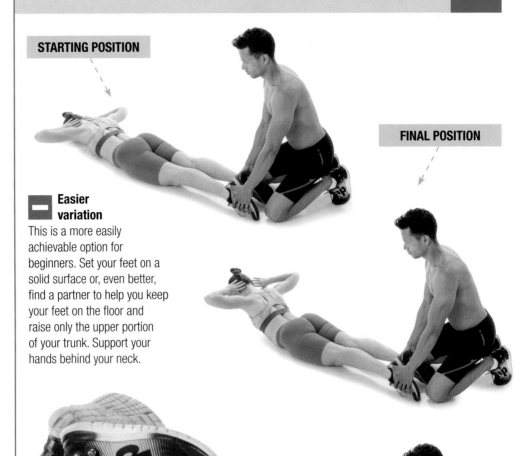

STARTING POSITION

FINAL POSITION

▬ Easier variation

This is a more easily achievable option for beginners. Set your feet on a solid surface or, even better, find a partner to help you keep your feet on the floor and raise only the upper portion of your trunk. Support your hands behind your neck.

STARTING POSITION

✚ Harder variation

If you prefer to increase the intensity, you can do a simple arch with a weight. To do this, find a partner to hold down your feet or set them so that they do not rise.
Hold a weight with both hands in front of your head, and complete the arch, raising the upper portion of your trunk and lifting the weight. You can use the same water jug as in other exercises, and fill it more as you gain strength.

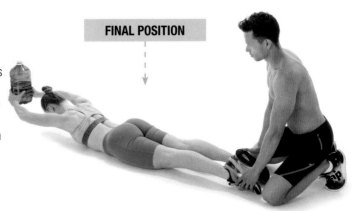

FINAL POSITION

17 Inverted Shoulder Press

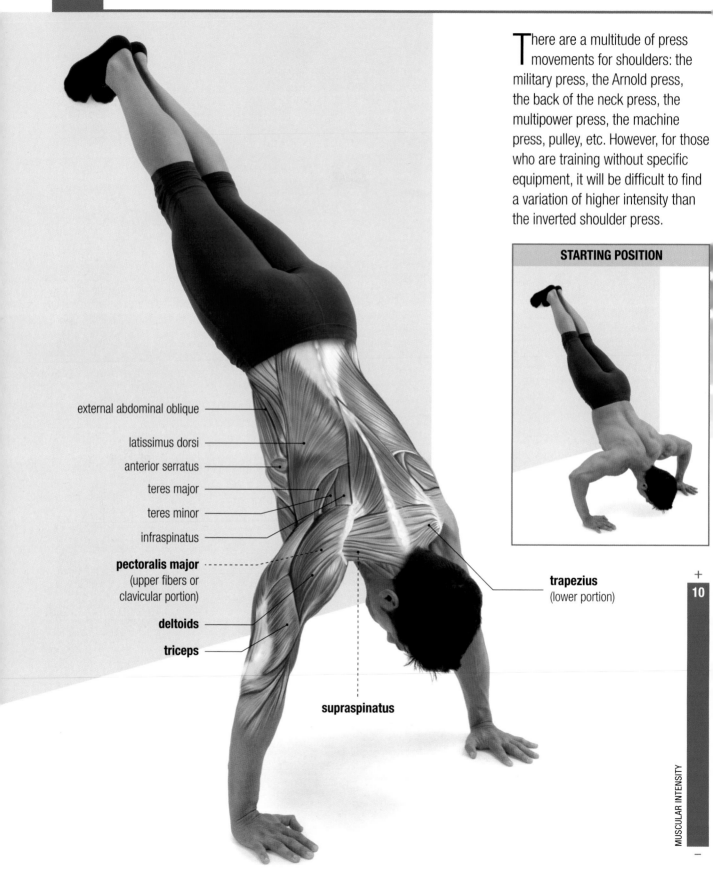

There are a multitude of press movements for shoulders: the military press, the Arnold press, the back of the neck press, the multipower press, the machine press, pulley, etc. However, for those who are training without specific equipment, it will be difficult to find a variation of higher intensity than the inverted shoulder press.

STARTING POSITION

external abdominal oblique

latissimus dorsi

anterior serratus

teres major

teres minor

infraspinatus

pectoralis major
(upper fibers or
clavicular portion)

deltoids

triceps

supraspinatus

trapezius
(lower portion)

+

10

MUSCULAR INTENSITY

−

ALTERNATIVE EXERCISES **17**

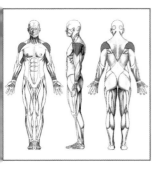

Execution

Get into an inverted vertical position, facing a wall and supported on your hands. In order to attain this position, first put the palms of your hands on the floor and progressively move your feet up the wall. Once you are in vertical position, flex your elbows and move downward, moving your head toward the floor. Then extend your elbows and raise up again.

Technical considerations

- Keep your trunk and lower extremities aligned.

- Be sure that your hand support is stable.

- The more vertical your position, the greater the work for your deltoids and the less work for the pectorals.

➖ Easier variation

For beginning bodybuilding athletes, a more accessible and effective alternative are known as *shoulder push-ups*. This exercise is done with the hips flexed, so as to allow the upper half of the body to be in an almost vertical position while the feet are on the floor, thus providing greater stability and reducing the difficulty.

FINAL POSITION

STARTING POSITION

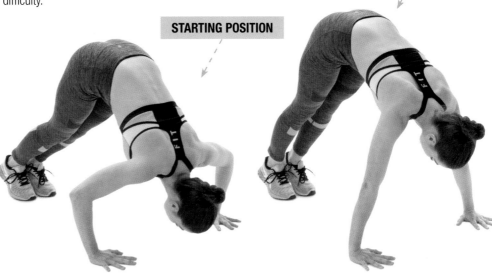

STARTING POSITION

➕ Harder variation

Supporting your hands on a pair of elevated supports, such as wood blocks or books, will make it possible for you to lengthen the movement to descend further and, therefore, to increase the difficulty. Although the principal exercise is tremendously intense, this variation, when well executed, will further increase the challenge. This is only recommended for advanced athletes.

FINAL POSITION

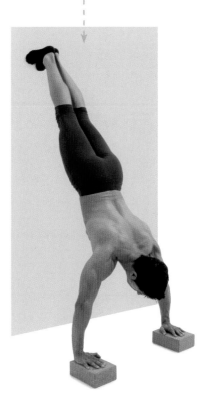

18 | **Overhead Press**

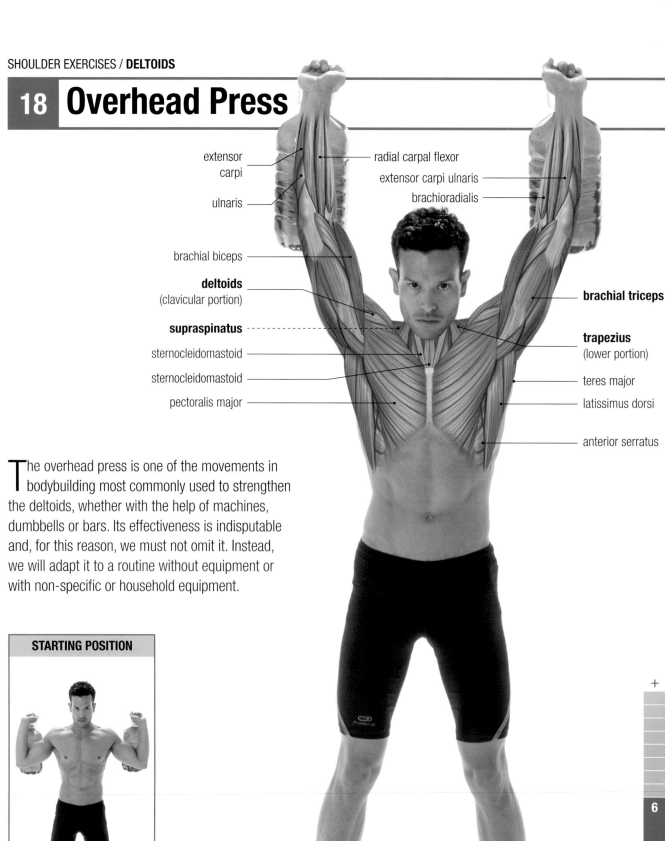

extensor carpi ulnaris

radial carpal flexor

extensor carpi ulnaris

brachioradialis

brachial biceps

deltoids
(clavicular portion)

supraspinatus

sternocleidomastoid

sternocleidomastoid

pectoralis major

brachial triceps

trapezius
(lower portion)

teres major

latissimus dorsi

anterior serratus

The overhead press is one of the movements in bodybuilding most commonly used to strengthen the deltoids, whether with the help of machines, dumbbells or bars. Its effectiveness is indisputable and, for this reason, we must not omit it. Instead, we will adapt it to a routine without equipment or with non-specific or household equipment.

STARTING POSITION

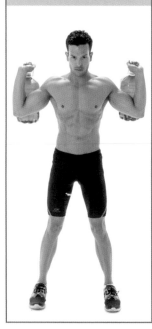

MUSCULAR INTENSITY

+

6

−

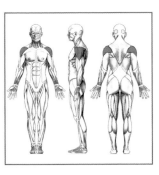

Execution

Hold a weight with each hand. Water jugs have the advantage of making it possible for you to regulate the weight by filling them to a greater or lesser degree. Their cost is also low. Flex your elbows and keep your hands up. From this position, extend your elbows, moving the water jugs upward as high as possible and making sure that your arms remain perpendicular to the ground.

Technical considerations

- Keep your back straight.

- If you are doing the exercise while standing, keep your knees slightly flexed.

- Be sure that your forearms remain perpendicular to the floor throughout the repetition.

▬ Easier variation

The same exercise can be executed with less weight and less technical difficulty, using only one item as a weight. Hold it in front of your chest with both hands and then raise it over your head. Repeat the cycle several times.

✚ Harder variation

In this variation, the degree of inclination determines the resistance that you apply (the greater the inclination, the greater the resistance). Nonetheless, the technical difficulty increases so that when hanging by a cord, it is more challenging to keep your balance and your body aligned.

STARTING POSITION

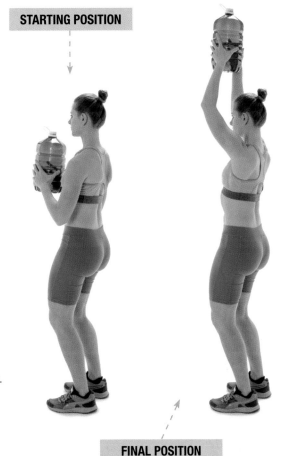

FINAL POSITION

STARTING POSITION

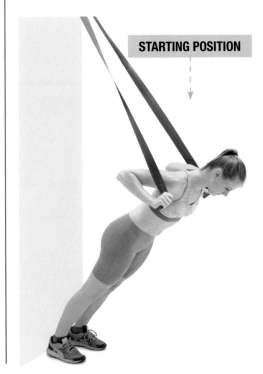

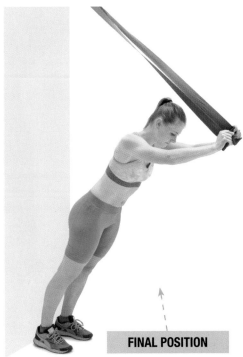

FINAL POSITION

19 | Front Incline Raise

Raises are bodybuilding movements that isolate the work to the deltoids very effectively. In overhead raises, this phenomenon is even more apparent, since the effort falls almost completely on the deltoids, particularly the anterior deltoids.

STARTING POSITION

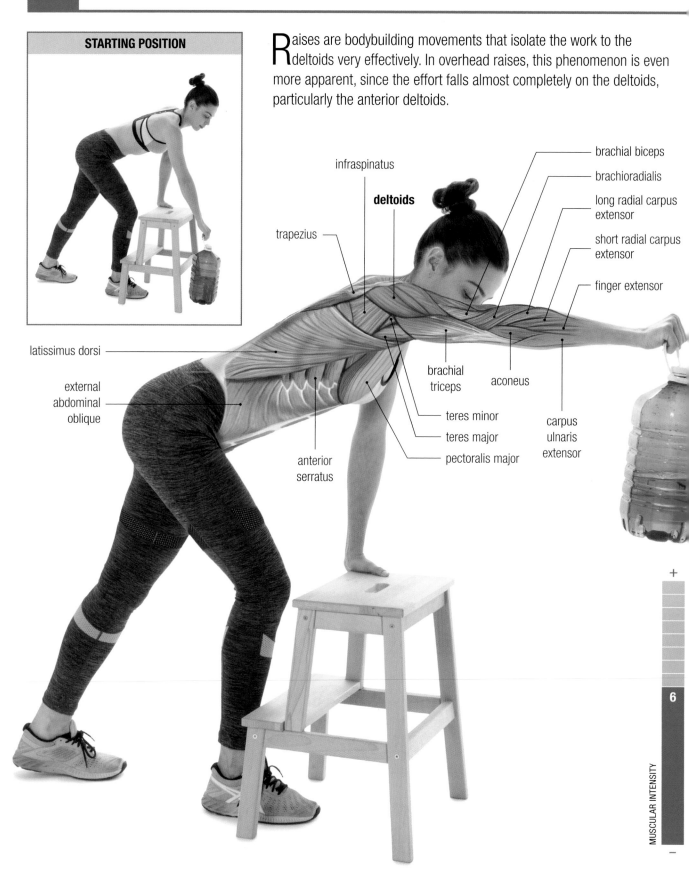

infraspinatus

trapezius

deltoids

brachial biceps

brachioradialis

long radial carpus extensor

short radial carpus extensor

finger extensor

latissimus dorsi

external abdominal oblique

brachial triceps

aconeus

teres minor

teres major

anterior serratus

pectoralis major

carpus ulnaris extensor

MUSCULAR INTENSITY

6

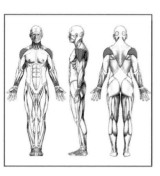

Execution

Support one hand on a chair, bench or low table, so that your trunk is inclined forward, almost parallel to the floor. With the other hand, hold an item that can be used as a weight. The water jug is a very versatile item, but any other object will also work. Raise the water jug forward without changing the position of your elbow.

Technical considerations

- Your supporting arm must have its elbow slightly flexed in order to cushion you during the movement.

- The elbow of the working arm must also be slightly flexed, to protect the joint.

- Your back must remain straight.

▬ Easier variation

Pass the nylon belt through an elevated support and hold one end with each hand. Allow yourself to hang backward slightly and by raising your hands, pull on the ends of the belt, trying to pull yourself back to a vertical position. This variation, with a little inclination, provides good results with a lesser degree of difficulty.

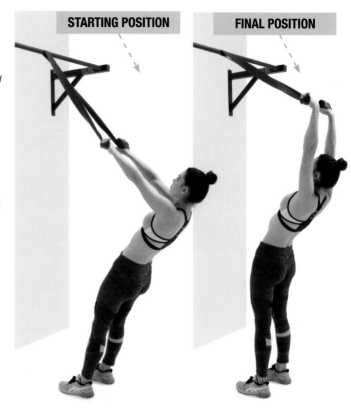

STARTING POSITION   FINAL POSITION

✚ Harder variation

Execute the same process as in variation 1, but increase the body's incline at the beginning, which will thus increase the difficulty. As you increase the incline, the execution will be more difficult and become impossible at not very pronounced angles, given the low participation of other muscle groups.

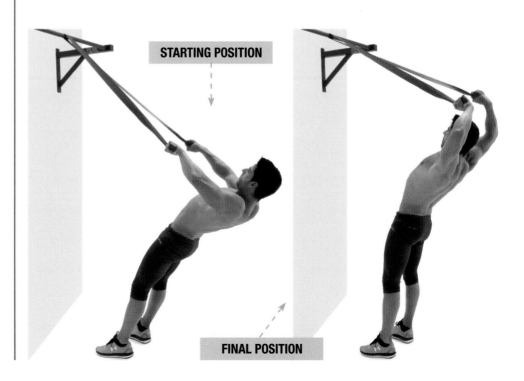

STARTING POSITION

FINAL POSITION

20 | Shoulder Extensions

This classic bodybuilding exercise makes it possible to develop the deltoids, especially their posterior portion. It also contributes to strengthening the external shoulder rotators, so that, with small adaptations, it must be a mandatory part of the repertory of any athlete of this discipline.

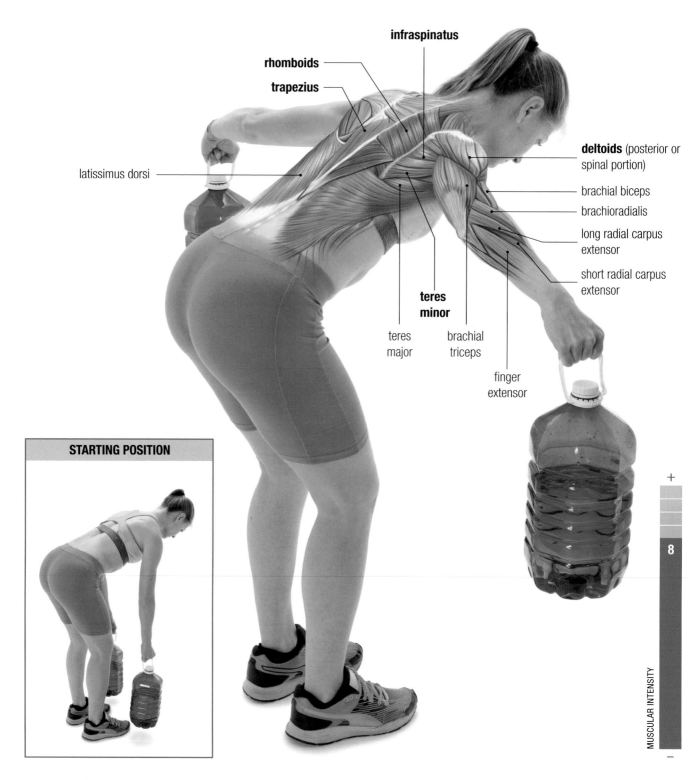

infraspinatus

rhomboids

trapezius

latissimus dorsi

deltoids (posterior or spinal portion)

brachial biceps

brachioradialis

long radial carpus extensor

short radial carpus extensor

teres minor

teres major

brachial triceps

finger extensor

STARTING POSITION

MUSCULAR INTENSITY

+

8

−

ALTERNATIVE EXERCISES **20**

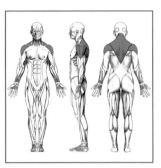

Technical considerations

- Be sure that your back remains straight and does not curve.

- Keep your knees flexed.

- Avoid flexing your elbows excessively.

Execution

Hold a weight in each hand, making sure that this weight is the same for both hands. Water jugs are a good option since they make degrees of resistance possible and are low cost items. Lean your trunk forward, slightly flex your knees, and with your back straight, raise the water jugs at both sides of the body, keeping a slight flexion in your elbows.

➖ Easier variation

If you want a variation with less difficulty, execute the same work in suspension. Grab both ends of the belt, previously connected to an elevated support, and put one foot behind the other.
The body's back incline will be slight. Open your arms, raising your hands toward your sides and return your body to a vertical position.

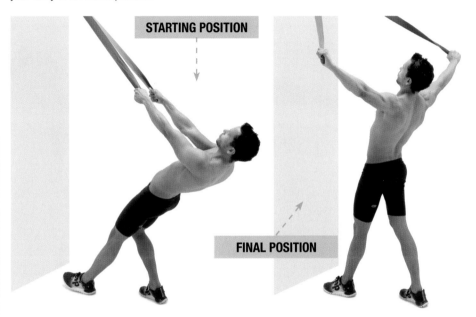

STARTING POSITION

FINAL POSITION

➕ Harder variation

In order to increase resistance and difficulty, it is sufficient to modify the previous exercise. Place your feet next to each other and increase the incline of your body, so that you are hanging by the belts. Open your arms again, trying to raise your trunk. To change the difficulty of the exercise, you can increase or decrease the incline of the body.

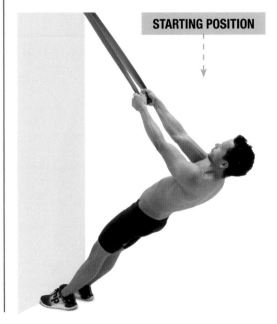

STARTING POSITION

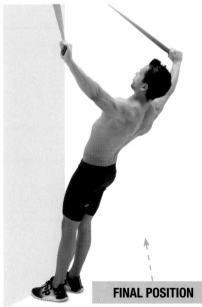

FINAL POSITION

21 | **Lateral Raises**

Raises are used to facilitate the development of the deltoids. Specifically, lateral raises, which are the most used exercises in bodybuilding gyms, are ideal for strengthening this muscle group, especially the acromial portion.

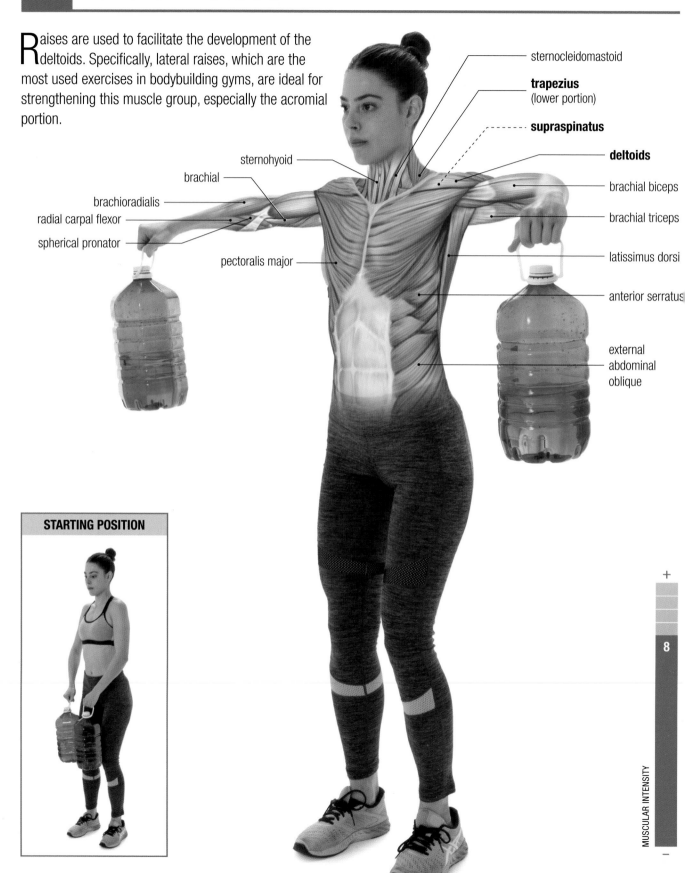

sternocleidomastoid

trapezius
(lower portion)

supraspinatus

deltoids

brachial biceps

brachial triceps

latissimus dorsi

anterior serratus

external
abdominal
oblique

sternohyoid

brachial

brachioradialis

radial carpal flexor

spherical pronator

pectoralis major

STARTING POSITION

MUSCULAR INTENSITY

+

8

−

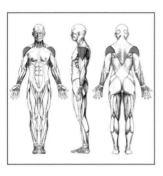

Execution

Hold a weight with each hand in front of your body, allowing it to hang, but keeping a certain degree of flexion in your elbows. Raise your hands toward your sides until your arms form a cross, without varying the flexion of your elbows. At the highest point of the repetition, your shoulders should be at a 90-degree angle. Lower the weight again and repeat the process.

Technical considerations

- Keep your elbows slightly flexed from the beginning to the end of the repetition.

- Your knees should be slightly flexed during the entire execution to cushion the movements of the weights and not injure your back.

- In order to protect your shoulders, it is preferable for your elbows to not exceed the height of the shoulders at the highest part of the exercise.

 Easier variation

With the same weights, and starting from the same initial position, flex your elbows and try to move the backs of your hands to your chin, keeping your shoulders high. This exercise, called an upright row, will enable you to work the deltoids with a lesser intensity than that of the principal exercise.

Harder variation

This variation is ideal for those who train with a partner. The function of the partner consists of providing resistance to the movement, increasing it as a function of the abilities of the person doing the exercise. Remember that your elbows must be at 90 degrees and your partner will put pressure on them with the palms of his hands to provide resistance.

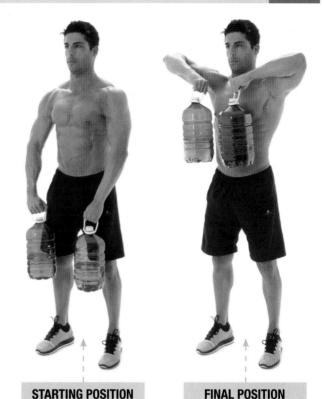

STARTING POSITION

FINAL POSITION

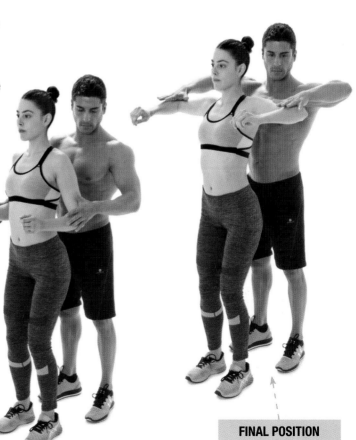

STARTING POSITION

FINAL POSITION

22 | **Front raises**

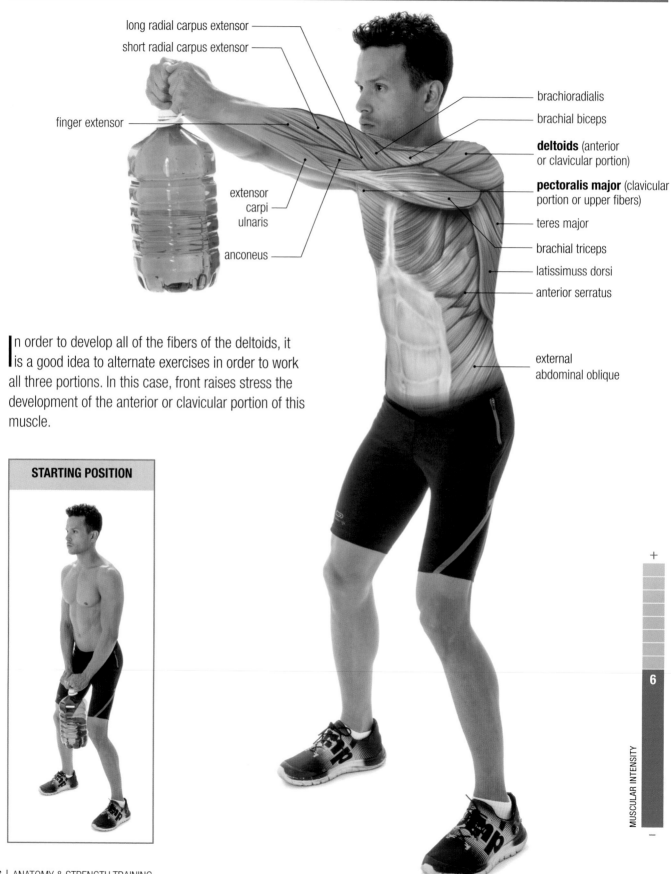

long radial carpus extensor

short radial carpus extensor

finger extensor

extensor carpi ulnaris

anconeus

brachioradialis

brachial biceps

deltoids (anterior or clavicular portion)

pectoralis major (clavicular portion or upper fibers)

teres major

brachial triceps

latissimuss dorsi

anterior serratus

external abdominal oblique

In order to develop all of the fibers of the deltoids, it is a good idea to alternate exercises in order to work all three portions. In this case, front raises stress the development of the anterior or clavicular portion of this muscle.

STARTING POSITION

MUSCULAR INTENSITY

+

6

−

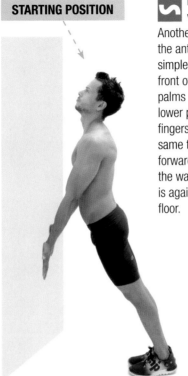

Execution

Hold a weight with both hands, so that it is hanging in front of you.

We use a water jug because of its wonderful versatility, but any other item with similar characteristics will also work. Your elbows should be almost completely extended, your back straight and your knees slightly flexed. Flex your shoulders and raise the object in front of you until your hands are in front of your face.

Technical considerations

- Remember to keep your knees slightly flexed and your back straight to protect the lumbar area.

- Keep your elbows completely extended.

- When your hands are in front of your face, stop the upward motion.

STARTING POSITION

Easier variation

Another valid option for working the anterior deltoids is this simple wall exercise. Stand in front of a wall and place the palms of your hands on the lower portion of it, with your fingers pointed down, at the same time as you lean slightly forward. Slide your palms over the wall, upward, until your body is again perpendicular to the floor.

FINAL POSITION

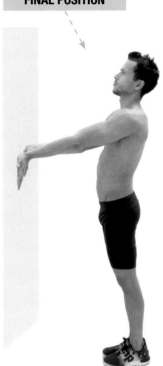

STARTING POSITION　　**FINAL POSITION**

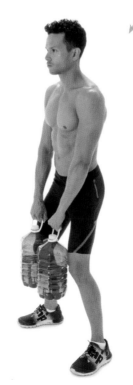

Harder variation

Adding difficulty to the principal exercise is as simple as adding resistance. Using a heavier object, or holding an object in each hand, and raising them, will give you the added difficulty which you will need over time. Water jugs are an excellent tool because they make it possible for us to vary the weight.

23 Resistance Curl With Foot

The curl movement which involves flexing the elbow, along with supination of the forearm, is, without a doubt, the exercise that achieves the greatest activation of the brachial biceps. Finding options like this one, which make it possible for us to execute it with resistance but without specific equipment, will make it possible to put together a powerful routine for the arms, wherever we are.

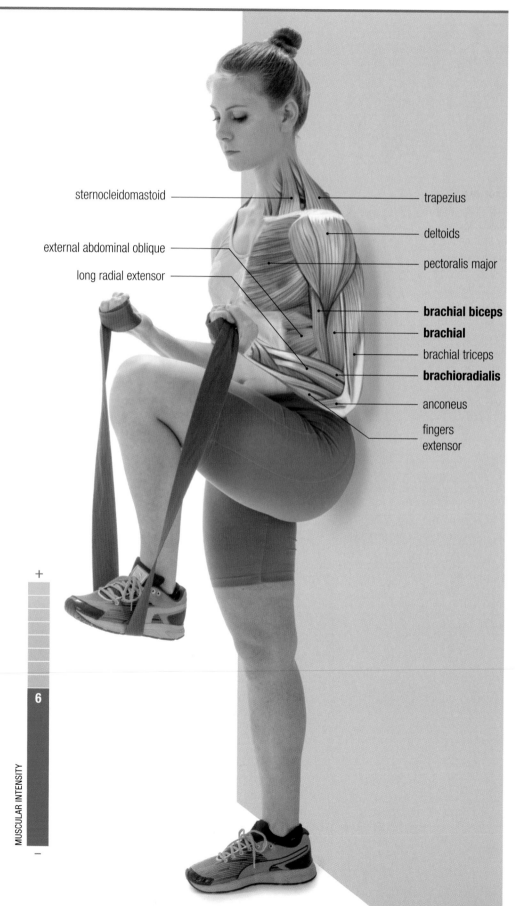

sternocleidomastoid

trapezius

deltoids

external abdominal oblique

pectoralis major

long radial extensor

brachial biceps

brachial

brachial triceps

brachioradialis

anconeus

fingers extensor

STARTING POSITION

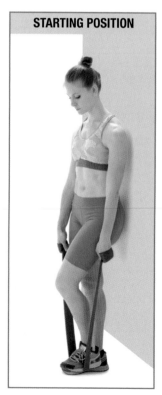

+

6

−

MUSCULAR INTENSITY

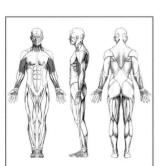

Execution

Support your back against a wall, hold a belt in your hands by both ends and pass it under one foot. You can use a nylon belt, as shown in the figure, an elastic belt, a towel or another similar object. In the starting position, the foot must almost be on the floor and the elbows extended. Flex your elbows as the same time as you move your forearms to supination. With your foot, apply the appropriate resistance.

Technical considerations

- Keep your elbows close to your trunk.

- Avoid using cords which may roll under the soles of your feet, and regulate the resistance with this.

- Keep your back supported by the wall.

 Easier variation

You can simplify the exercise by hanging a water jug from the center of the belt. This will provide you with scalable, although always reduced, resistance, and will enable you to support yourself on both feet, thus benefiting from more stability during execution. The movements of the elbows and forearms will be the same as in the principal exercise.

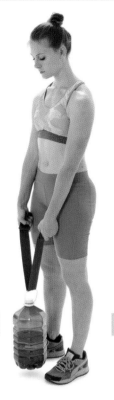

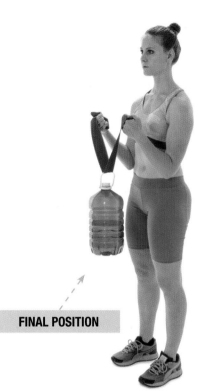

STARTING POSITION

FINAL POSITION

STARTING POSITION

FINAL POSITION

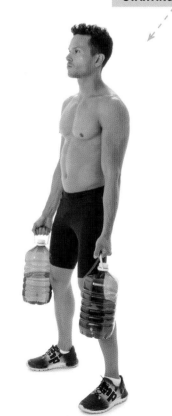

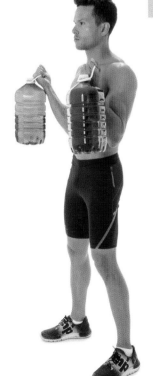

 Harder variation

In order to perform the next exercise, you will need two objects as weights. You should hold a weight in each hand and limit yourself to flexing your elbows in order to raise the weights. Water jugs will enable you to work with higher resistance, but will limit the pronation-supination movement.

24 Suspension Curls

Suspension exercises are very popular because they require little equipment and, in the majority of cases, are of alterable intensity. This is one of the exercises in suspension with which you will achieve greater increase in muscle mass. The raised position of the elbows provides a maximum contraction of the brachial biceps and an intense, burning sensation.

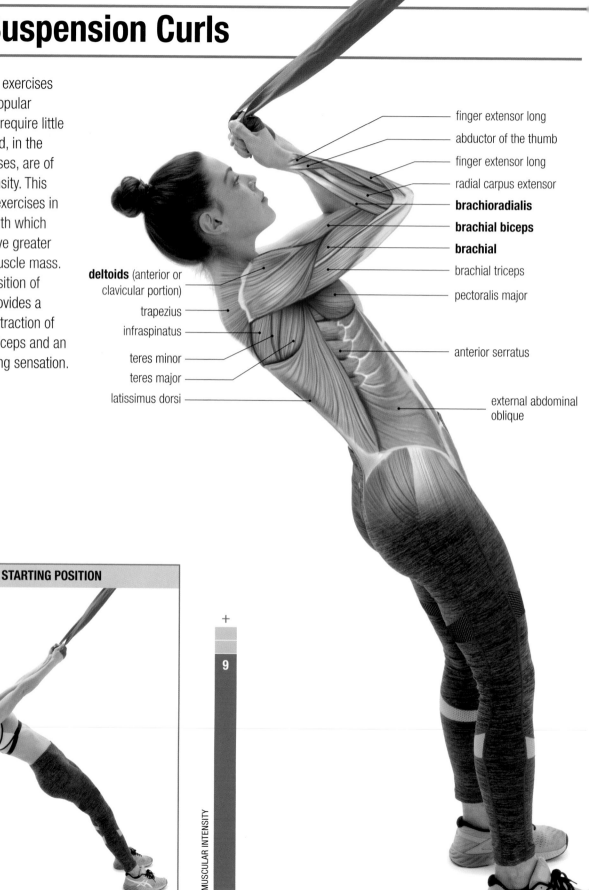

finger extensor long
abductor of the thumb
finger extensor long
radial carpus extensor
brachioradialis
brachial biceps
brachial
brachial triceps
pectoralis major
anterior serratus
external abdominal oblique

deltoids (anterior or clavicular portion)
trapezius
infraspinatus
teres minor
teres major
latissimus dorsi

STARTING POSITION

MUSCULAR INTENSITY

+
9
−

ALTERNATIVE EXERCISES 24

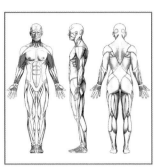

Execution
Pass a nylon or similar belt through a vertical support and hold one of its ends with each hand. Lean back until you are hanging, with your hands in front of you and your elbows extended. Without lowering your elbows from the point where they are flexed, lift your own weight and try to raise your fists to your forehead.

Technical considerations

■ Your shoulders must always remain in the same angle of flexion.

■ Try to raise your fists toward your forehead, keeping your neck straight.

■ Remember that by regulating the inclination of your body, you will regulate the intensity of the exercise.

➖ Easier variation
If you put a weight on the belt so that it is suspended on the other side of the support, you will be able to do the same movement as in the original exercise, but while remaining standing. The bodybuilding movement will continue to be effective, but you will work with the weight at a lower intensity.

➕ Harder variation
By increasing the inclination of your body at the starting position, you will be able to increase the difficulty of the exercise, all the way to impossible levels. This variation with greater inclination is only within the reach of advanced athletes, and those with good technique, with swelling and muscular exhaustion occurring after just a few repetitions.

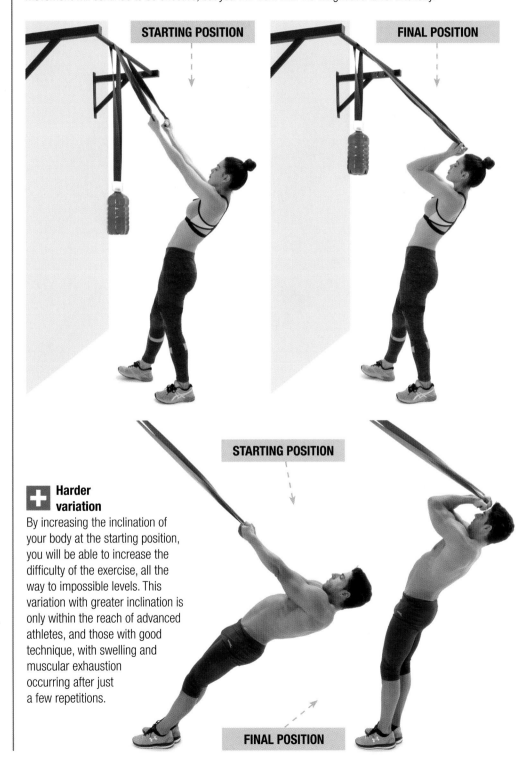

STARTING POSITION

FINAL POSITION

STARTING POSITION

FINAL POSITION

25 Fixed Bar Suspended Curls

Substituting weights for our body weight is always an alternative when training without specific equipment. It is a bit unusual to see this in working the brachial biceps. Nonetheless, suspended curls that are properly executed are incredibly effective and the muscle mass increase that they provide is difficult to equal.

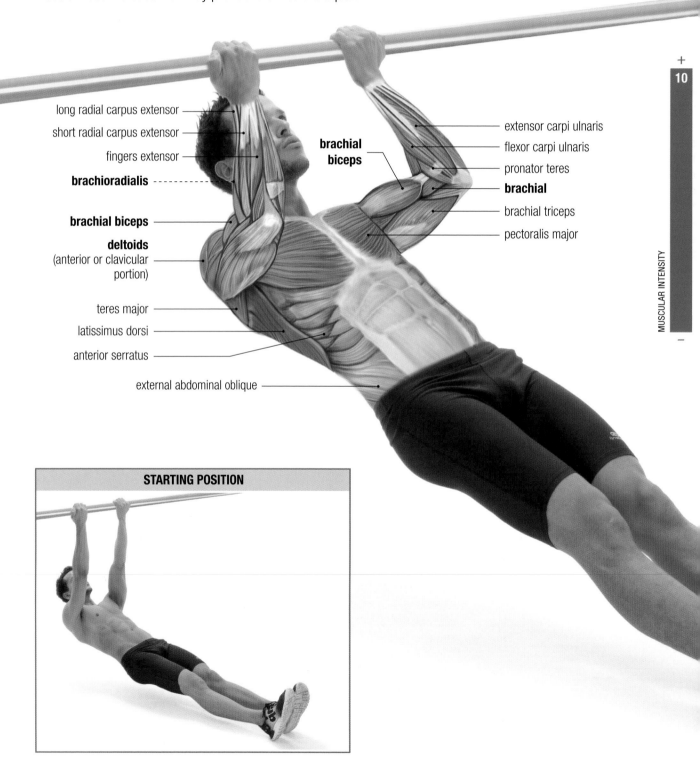

long radial carpus extensor
short radial carpus extensor
fingers extensor
brachioradialis

brachial biceps
deltoids
(anterior or clavicular portion)

teres major
latissimus dorsi
anterior serratus

external abdominal oblique

brachial biceps

extensor carpi ulnaris
flexor carpi ulnaris
pronator teres
brachial
brachial triceps
pectoralis major

+
10

MUSCULAR INTENSITY

–

STARTING POSITION

ALTERNATIVE EXERCISES   **25**

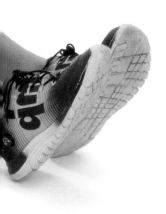

Execution

You will need a low, horizontal support, such as a railing or a strong table. Hold it with both hands in a supine grip and extend your arms such that you are hanging, head up, beneath the support, with your trunk and legs perfectly aligned. Flex your elbows and try to move your forehead close to the support.

Technical considerations

- Be certain to bring your forehead close to the horizontal support and not your chest, which would be the natural tendency.

- Keep your trunk and lower extremities perfectly aligned.

- Avoid too much of a gap between your elbows.

➖ Easier variation

Given the elevated difficulty of the principal exercise, new athletes can execute a body-weight curl. To do this, it is sufficient to hold one wrist with the opposite hand. Slowly flex the elbow of the wrist that is held by the opposite hand, push downward, making the task more difficult.

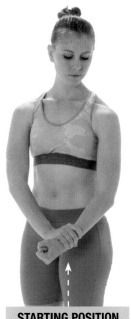

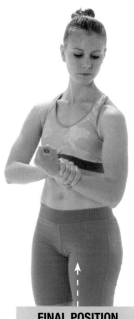

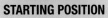

STARTING POSITION   **FINAL POSITION**

STARTING POSITION

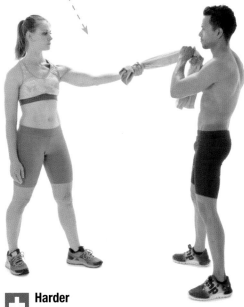

FINAL POSITION

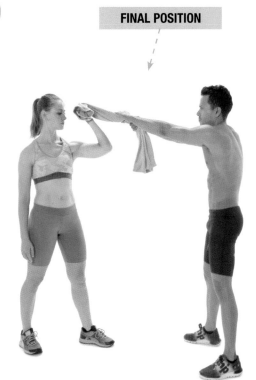

➕ Harder variation

This alternative exercise enables you to set the intensity to an appropriate level. Extend one arm in front of you and grasp the end of a towel, belt or similar object, in a supine position. A training partner should grasp the opposite end. Flex your elbow, trying to move your fist forward toward your forehead while your partner applies the desired resistance. If you prefer, you can do the exercise alone, using an elastic band anchored to a fixed point.

26 Vertical Extensions With Weight

Extending the elbow is the primordial function of the brachial triceps, but its long head is also a shoulder extensor. To do this, exercises executed with the elbow raised begin from a pre-stretched position of this muscle which makes them more difficult.

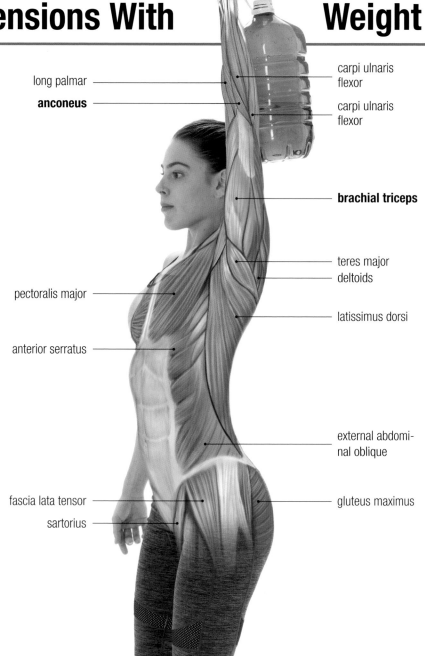

long palmar

anconeus

carpi ulnaris flexor

carpi ulnaris flexor

brachial triceps

teres major

deltoids

latissimus dorsi

pectoralis major

anterior serratus

external abdominal oblique

gluteus maximus

fascia lata tensor

sartorius

STARTING POSITION

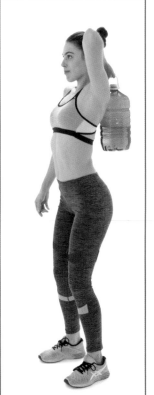

+

6

MUSCULAR INTENSITY

–

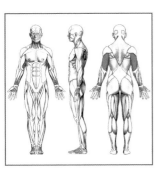

Execution

Beginning from a standing position, and keeping in mind that for standing exercises you must always keep your knees slightly flexed, grasp a weight with your hands and locate it behind your neck or back, depending on its length. Your elbow will remain flexed and close to your head. Extend your elbow, keeping it close to your head so that it lifts the weight.

Technical considerations

■ Your arm will stay almost perpendicular to the floor throughout the repetition.

■ The position of your shoulder must not vary.

■ Remember to keep both knees slightly flexed for cushioning to protect your lumbar spine.

■ Easier variation

With only a piece of a belt, towel or cord, you can do the same exercise with both arms at the same time. To do this, pass the cord through the handle of the water jug and hold an end in each hand so that it is hanging behind your back. Extend and flex your elbows in succession in order to move the weight.

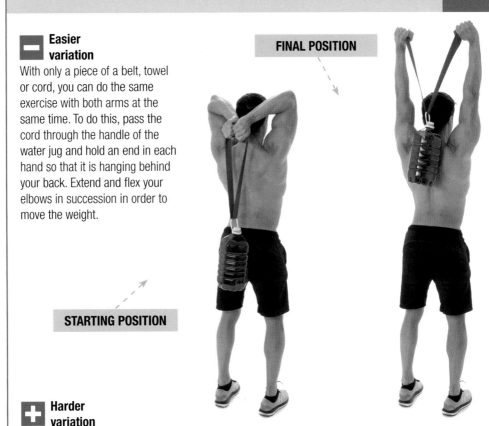

FINAL POSITION

STARTING POSITION

✛ Harder variation

If you are training with a partner and you have a piece of cord, towel or belt, you can work against your partner's resistance. Hold the cord by both ends while your partner, standing behind you, holds it by its center and pulls on it to stop your movement.

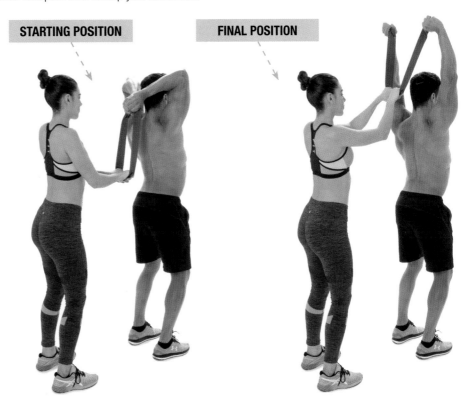

STARTING POSITION

FINAL POSITION

27 Diamond Push-Ups

This is one of the multiple variations on classic flexes. This time, the diamond flex, or flex with hands together, enables you to activate the work of your triceps with a small variation in the hand support and without the need for any auxiliary item. It is enough to use your body weight.

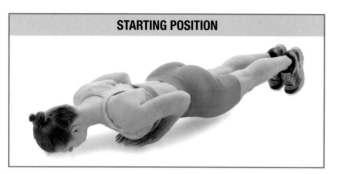

STARTING POSITION

Execution

Put yourself in a flexed position, but move your hands together so that your thumbs touch each other. You can also accomplish the support so that the tips of your thumbs and index fingers touch each other, forming a rhombus. At the lowest point of the exercise, your elbows will be flexed and your chest will be just over your hands. Extend your elbows and lift your trunk.

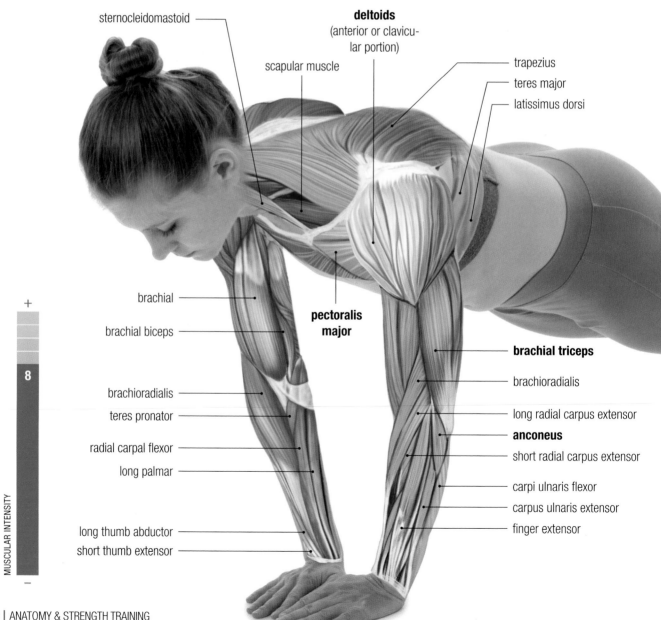

sternocleidomastoid

deltoids
(anterior or clavicular portion)

scapular muscle

trapezius

teres major

latissimus dorsi

brachial

brachial biceps

pectoralis major

brachial triceps

brachioradialis

brachioradialis

teres pronator

long radial carpus extensor

radial carpal flexor

anconeus

long palmar

short radial carpus extensor

carpi ulnaris flexor

carpus ulnaris extensor

finger extensor

long thumb abductor

short thumb extensor

MUSCULAR INTENSITY

+

8

−

ALTERNATIVE EXERCISES 27

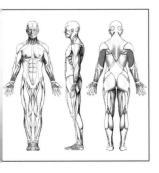

Technical considerations

- Keep your elbows pressed to your body at the beginning and as close together as possible, at the end of the movement.

- Be sure that your trunk and lower extremities are aligned at all times.

- Your hands must be together, but on the other hand, a small separation between your feet will provide you with greater stability.

➖ Easier variation

In an exercise that moves body weight with the upper body, adding inclination makes the exercise more difficult and decreasing inclination makes it easier. Standing, and supporting your hands on the wall, you can perform a simpler version of the diamond flexion. At the beginning, your body is inclined forward and, by extending your elbows, you will become perpendicular to the floor.

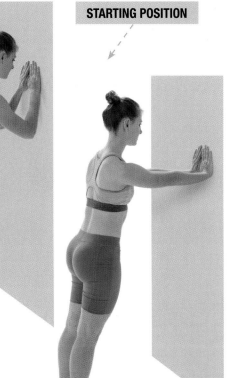

STARTING POSITION

FINAL POSITION

➕ Harder variation

You can add intensity to the diamond push-up if you seek the help of a partner. Your partner should push on your back with a hand or foot, preferably in the upper area and between your shoulder blades to minimize the risk of injury. Another alternative consists of doing the exercise with a backpack filled with books or other heavy items.

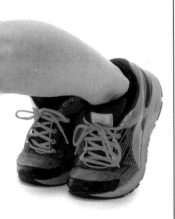

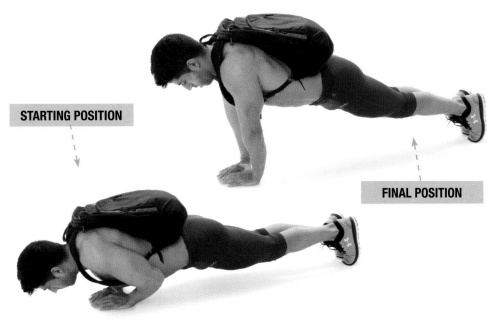

STARTING POSITION

FINAL POSITION

28 | Triceps Dips

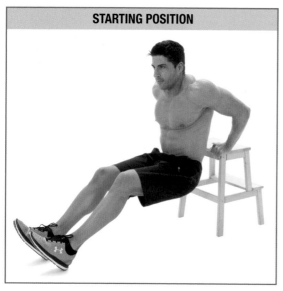

STARTING POSITION

Dip exercises work both the pectorals and the triceps, and even the anterior deltoids. The greater incidence on one or the other depends on the inclination of the trunk, the width of the grip and the location of the hands in relation to the body. Playing with these elements modifies the percentage of work for each muscle, without completely eliminating the participation of any of them.

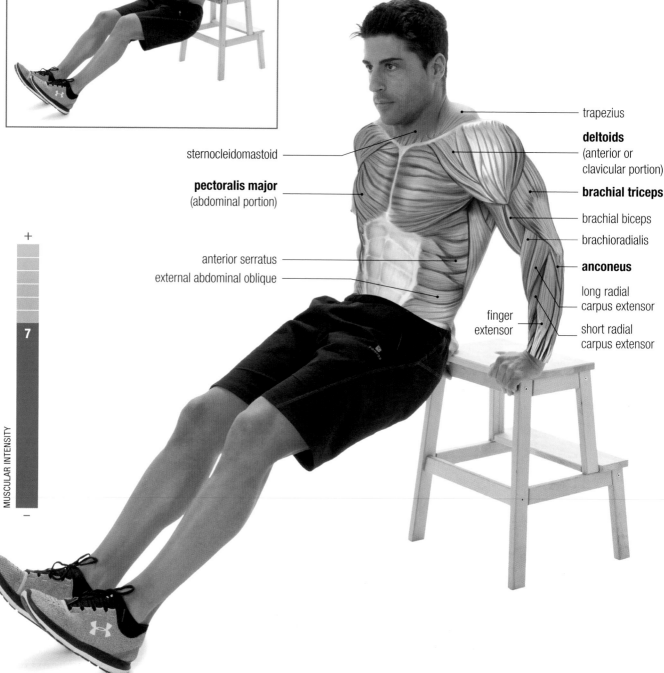

trapezius

deltoids
(anterior or clavicular portion)

sternocleidomastoid

pectoralis major
(abdominal portion)

brachial triceps

brachial biceps

brachioradialis

anterior serratus

anconeus

external abdominal oblique

long radial carpus extensor

finger extensor

short radial carpus extensor

MUSCULAR INTENSITY

+

7

−

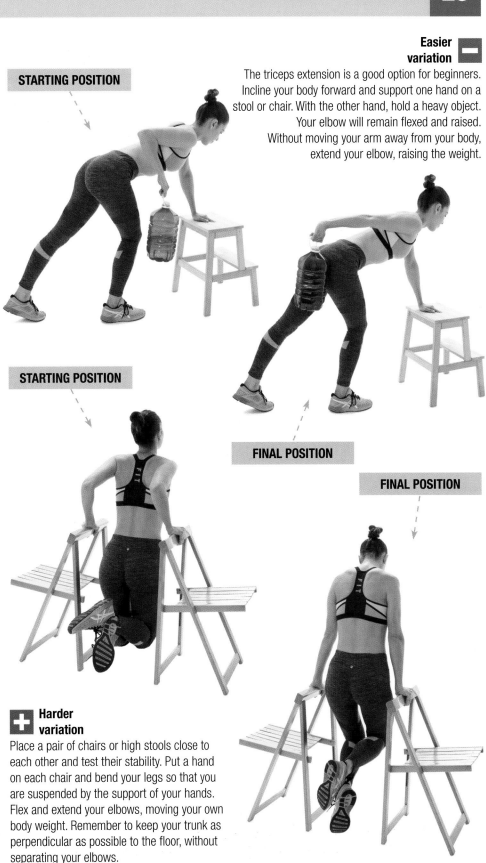

STARTING POSITION

Easier variation ▬

The triceps extension is a good option for beginners. Incline your body forward and support one hand on a stool or chair. With the other hand, hold a heavy object. Your elbow will remain flexed and raised. Without moving your arm away from your body, extend your elbow, raising the weight.

STARTING POSITION

FINAL POSITION

FINAL POSITION

Execution

Put a high stool or chair with its back toward you. Support yourself with both hands and put your legs forward, so that your arms support the largest portion of your weight. Flex your elbows, lowering your body and, when you reach the end of the repetition, extend them again, bearing your own weight while raising.

Technical considerations

■ Your hands must be supported relatively close.

■ Be sure that both elbows are as close as possible to each other throughout the repetition. Do not separate them.

■ Your feet will be supported on your ankles and your hip will remain separated from the bench so that you do not hit it on the back of the bench during the repetition.

Harder variation ✚

Place a pair of chairs or high stools close to each other and test their stability. Put a hand on each chair and bend your legs so that you are suspended by the support of your hands. Flex and extend your elbows, moving your own body weight. Remember to keep your trunk as perpendicular as possible to the floor, without separating your elbows.

29 Suspension Triceps Extensions

This time, we will the suspension trainer to work the triceps. We start from a stretched, or intermediate, position, similar to that used in a lying triceps extension with your back to the device. This pre-stretched position adds difficulty to the exercise, making it both tremendously effective and demanding.

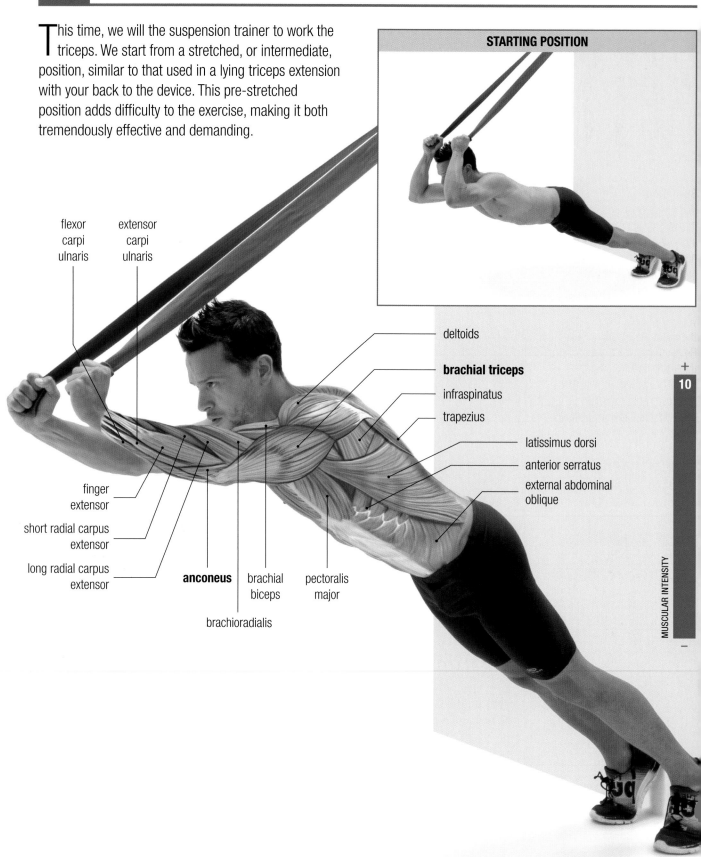

STARTING POSITION

flexor carpi ulnaris

extensor carpi ulnaris

deltoids

brachial triceps

infraspinatus

trapezius

latissimus dorsi

anterior serratus

external abdominal oblique

finger extensor

short radial carpus extensor

long radial carpus extensor

anconeus

brachial biceps

pectoralis major

brachioradialis

MUSCULAR INTENSITY

+
10
−

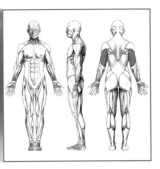

Execution

Pass a belt or a resistant cord through an elevated support such as a beam, a bar or a heavy tree branch. Grasp both ends of the belt with your hands and face your back to the support. Lean forward until you are suspended and find the appropriate inclination. Remember that, the greater the inclination, the greater the difficulty. Your elbows and shoulders will be flexed so that your hands are close to your head. Extend your elbows so that your body becomes increasingly perpendicular in relation to the ground.

Technical considerations

■ Keep your trunk and lower extremities aligned.

■ Try not to separate or open your elbows too much.

■ If you do this exercise often, supplement it with others that strengthen the external shoulder rotator muscles.

▬ Easier variation

With the same belt or cord, and support required for the principal exercise, you can also execute an exercise of less difficulty. Pass the belt through the support and hang a weight on its end. Grasp the other end with your back to the support and with one foot in front of the other. The arm holding the belt should be pointed toward your forehead, with the elbow flexed. Extend your elbow and move the weight upward as is also done by a pulley.

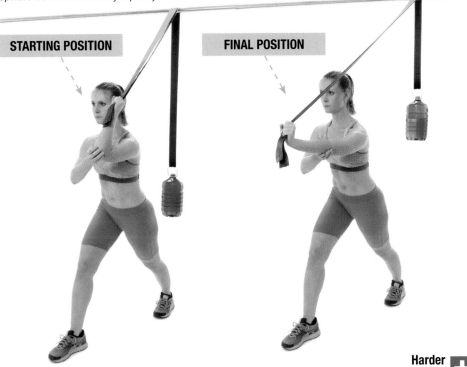

STARTING POSITION

FINAL POSITION

Harder variation ✚

Using a table or a railing or any other firm support as shown, you can execute an exercise similar to the principal exercise, but in your range of maximum difficulty. Lean toward the support and grasp it with both hands. Flex your elbows and remain hanging with your trunk and lower extremities aligned. Extend your elbows and also slightly extend your shoulders until your head is above the support.

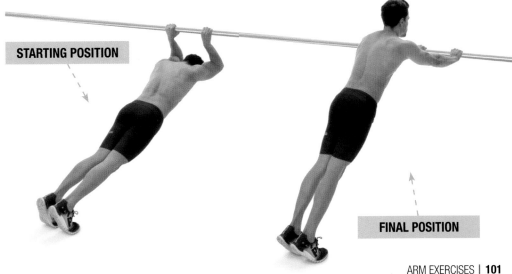

STARTING POSITION

FINAL POSITION

30 | **Plank**

The following exercise consists of working a muscle by an isometric contraction. This means that, as an exception, we contract it in a static position, without any movement, only maintaining the original position for several seconds, which requires great effort.

STATIC POSITION

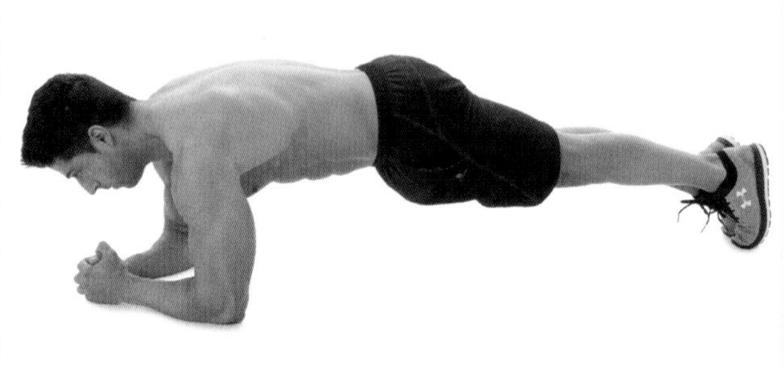

Execution

Lie facedown on the floor. Raise yourself on your toes and forearms, so that your trunk and lower extremities are aligned. In this position, the abdominal muscles make a significant effort to keep the body from arching downward. Hold this position for as much time as possible.

MUSCULAR INTENSITY

5

anterior serratus
teres major
teres minor
trapezius
deltoids
iliopsoas
latissimus dorsi
gluteus maximus
internal abdominal oblique
external abdominal oblique
rectus abdominus
brachial triceps
brachial biceps

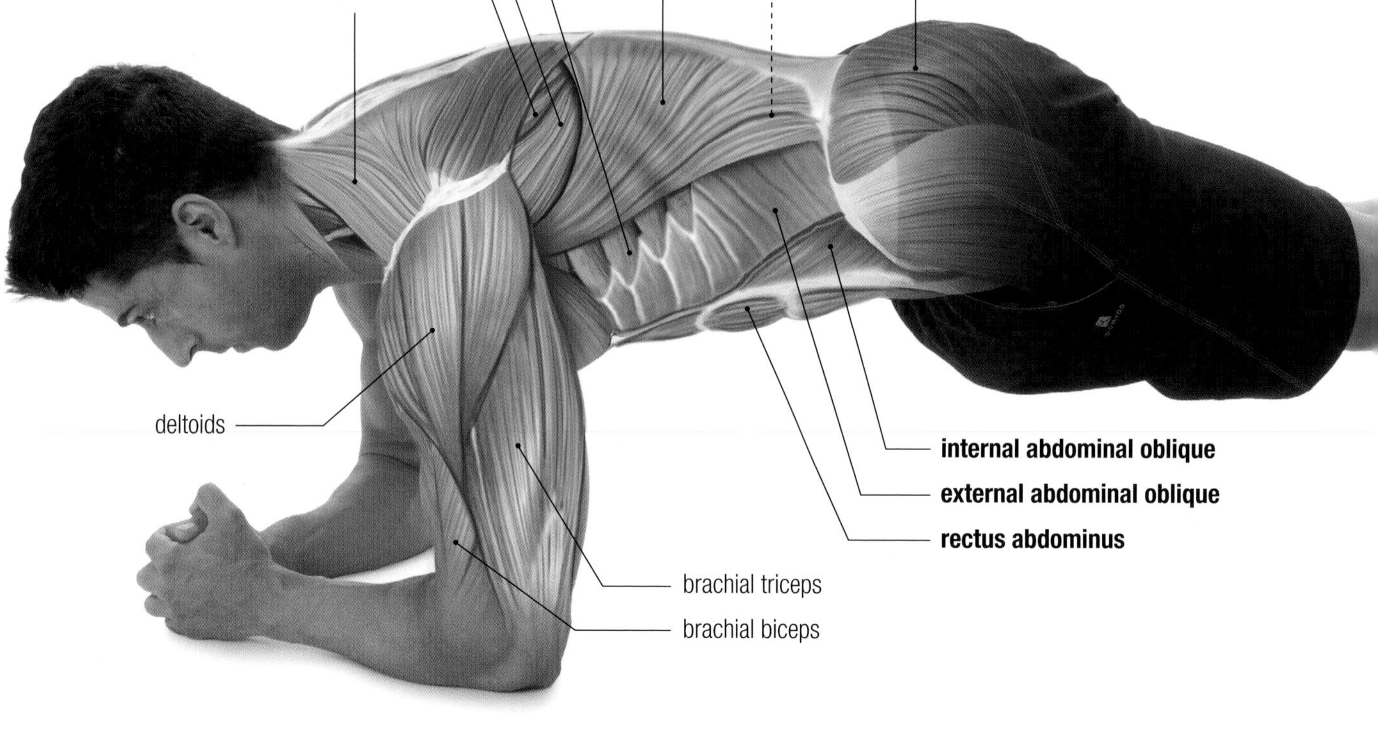

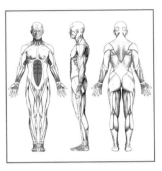

Technical considerations

- Try to keep your lower extremities and trunk in perfect alignment.

- Contract the abdominal musculature and avoid arching your body toward the ground.

 Easier variation

If the classic plank is too difficult for you, try the variant with knee support, since it is an effective option and much more accessible. The only thing to consider is substituting the support with your toes for support with your knees and the part of the thigh just above it.

STATIC POSITION

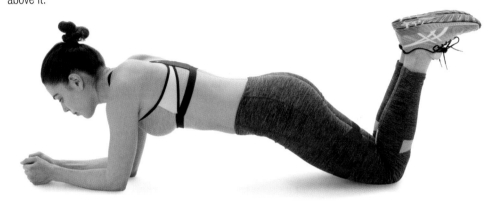

 Harder variation

In order to increase the degree of difficulty, you can add isometric contractions to the basic position. Start from a classic plank and execute small flexes of the trunk that add movement and intensity. It is important that the trunk arches upward when rising, but never downward when descending, with the lowest point being the classic plank position.

STARTING POSITION

FINAL POSITION

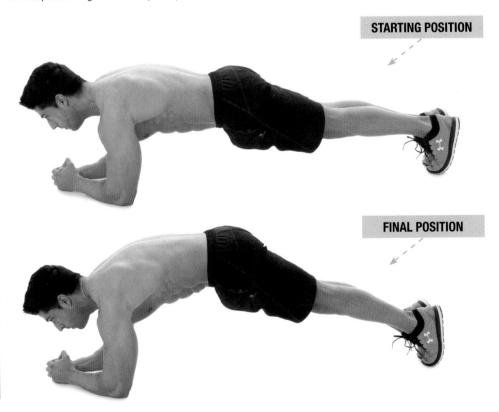

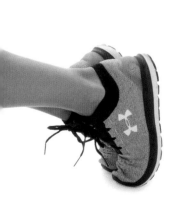

31 Crunch With Vertical Arms

Movements for working the abdominals are among the most popular, but are also commonly the worst executed, since they must be limited to a very short flex motion and, on the other hand, hip flexing is often prioritized. This simple, beginning exercise can be very useful in improving technique.

STARTING POSITION

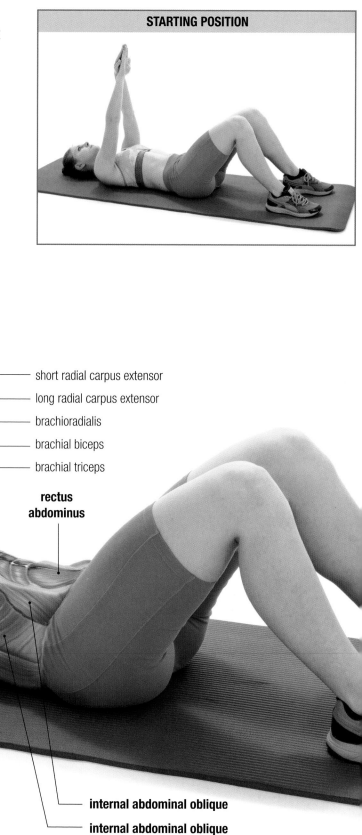

MUSCULAR INTENSITY

+

4

−

short radial carpus extensor

long radial carpus extensor

brachioradialis

brachial biceps

brachial triceps

rectus abdominus

anconeus

deltoids

teres minor

teres major

anterior serratus

pectoralis major

latissimus dorsi

internal abdominal oblique

internal abdominal oblique

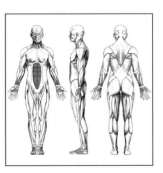

Technical considerations

■ Focus on working the abdominals.

■ Avoid moving your legs or flexing your hips once you have begun the exercise.

■ Limit the movement to a few centimeters.

Execution

Lie face-up with your hips and knees flexed. Point your arms up, one hand over the other, with your fingers pointing toward the ceiling. Execute a short flexing motion of the trunk for the purpose of separating the upper portion of the back from its support, and raise the ends of your fingers a few centimeters. After a few repetitions, or if you hold the final position for a few seconds, you will experience the effectiveness of the exercise, despite its static appearance.

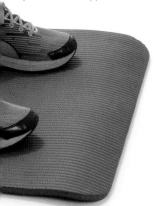

▬ Easier variation

This variation, with difficulty level similar to that of the principal exercise, will contribute to improving technique in the early days of training. Lie face-up, but with your hands positioned as in the traditional crunch. Although we often see the hands behind the neck, the best position is to put your fingers to your temples and avoid the temptation to pull on your neck because this could be harmful to the cervical spine area.

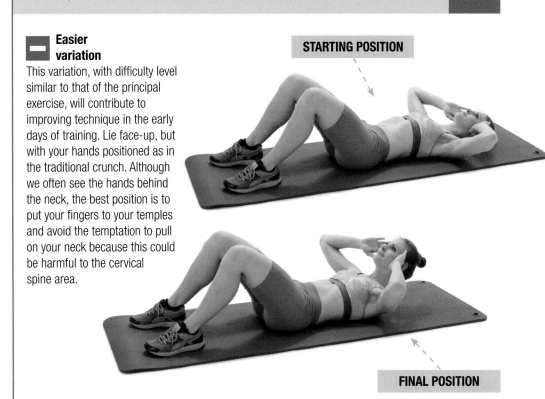

STARTING POSITION

FINAL POSITION

➕ Harder variation

The initial position for this exercise and the movement are identical, but we have added a weight to increase difficulty. With your arms extended toward the ceiling, hold a heavy item, such as a book, a bottle of water, a medicine ball or even the usual item, used for its versatility, the water jug. Try to raise it a few centimeters by flexing your trunk.

STARTING POSITION

FINAL POSITION

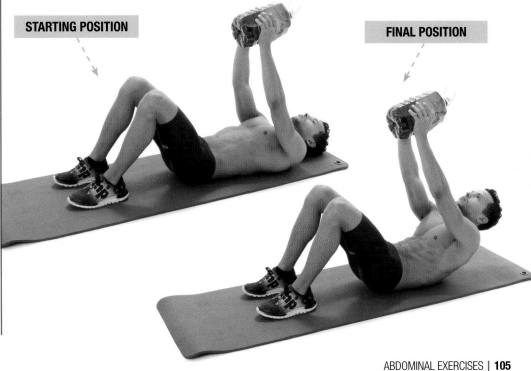

32 Hip Raises With Vertical Legs

The hip raise along with crunch movements is a bodybuilding exercise that is effective in the development of abdominal musculature. Both are based on flexing the trunk and only differ in the area that loses contact with the ground, or separates from it.

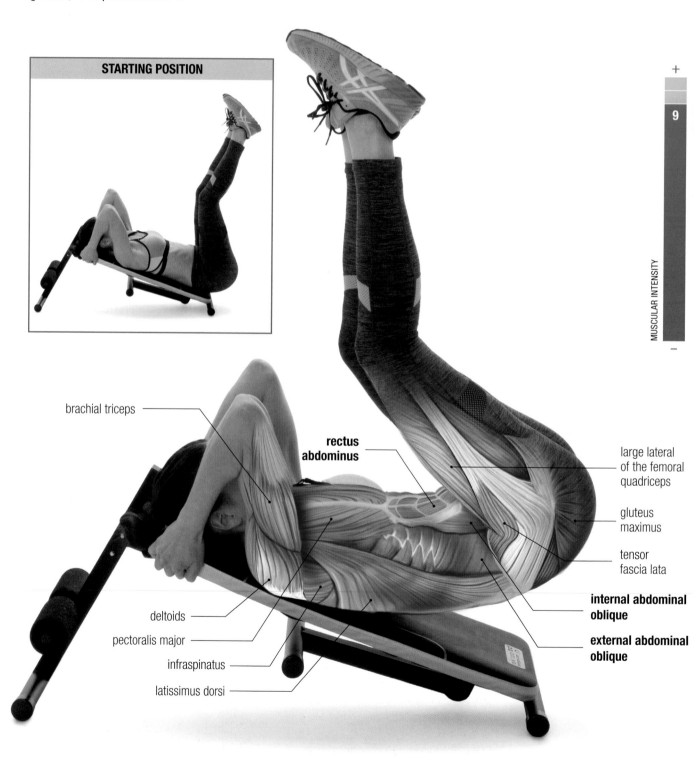

STARTING POSITION

MUSCULAR INTENSITY

+

9

−

brachial triceps

rectus
abdominus

large lateral
of the femoral
quadriceps

gluteus
maximus

tensor
fascia lata

deltoids

pectoralis major

infraspinatus

latissimus dorsi

internal abdominal
oblique

external abdominal
oblique

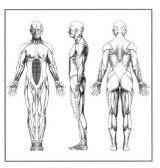

Execution

Lie face-up on an inclined bench. If you do not have one, you can put a chock on any flat surface such as a board. Your shoulders should be at the high end and your hips at the low end. Hold yourself to the bench with both hands and push your feet upward with your knees extended. Contract your abdominals and try to separate your hips and the lower portion of your back from the bench.

Technical considerations

- The objective is to separate your butt and the lower portion of your back from the bench, keeping the degree of hip flexing unvarying from the starting position.

- Use your hands to keep you from sliding.

- Avoid pulsing your lower extremities and execute the movement slowly.

Easier variation

You can do the same exercise on the ground or on a flat surface, which will decrease its difficulty. Raise your hips from the ground and try to raise your feet a bit higher than your starting position without moving them toward your head, and with the knees almost completely extended. A movement of the feet from 5 to 10 centimeters will be sufficient.

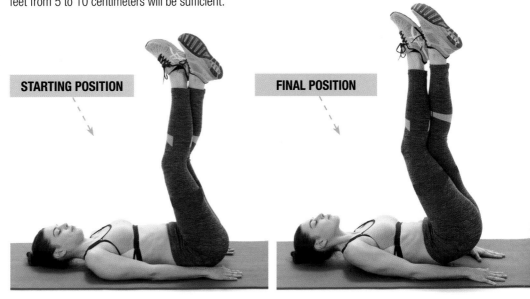

STARTING POSITION   FINAL POSITION

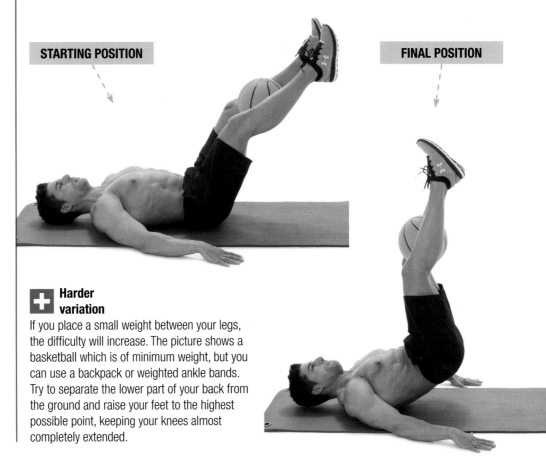

STARTING POSITION   FINAL POSITION

Harder variation

If you place a small weight between your legs, the difficulty will increase. The picture shows a basketball which is of minimum weight, but you can use a backpack or weighted ankle bands. Try to separate the lower part of your back from the ground and raise your feet to the highest possible point, keeping your knees almost completely extended.

33 | Incline Hip Raises

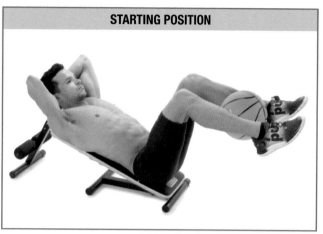

STARTING POSITION

A dding an incline to the elevation of the hips is an option that makes it possible to increase the difficulty of this bodybuilding movement. It is not important if your shoulders are lower than your hips, or vice versa. When executing a trunk flex with incline, the resistance and effectiveness of the exercise will be increased.

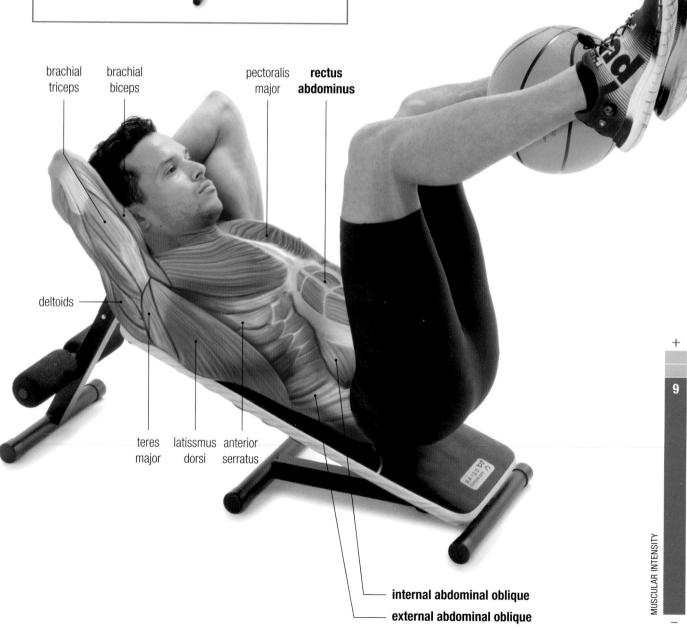

brachial triceps

brachial biceps

pectoralis major

rectus abdominus

deltoids

teres major

latissmus dorsi

anterior serratus

internal abdominal oblique

external abdominal oblique

MUSCULAR INTENSITY

+

9

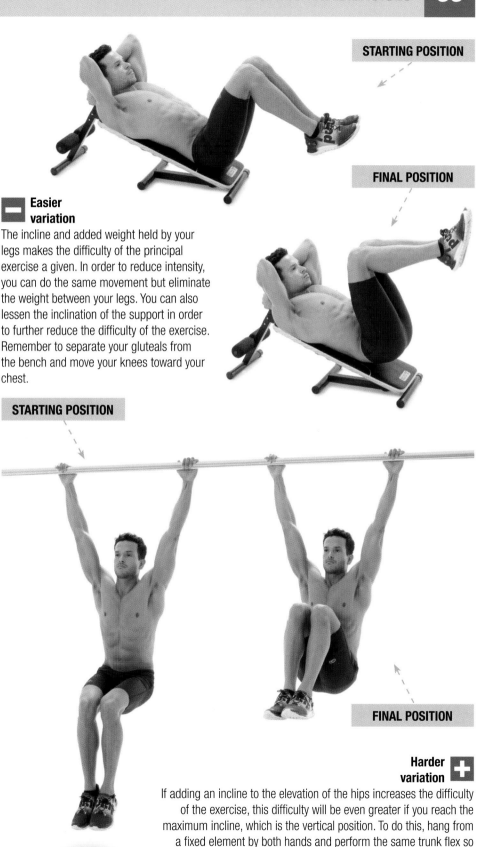

STARTING POSITION

FINAL POSITION

Execution

Lie face-up on an inclined surface, so that your hips are lower than your shoulders. You can use a bench, but any other flat surface can also be used if you put a chock under one end. Flex your hips and knees to 90 degrees and put an item between your legs that increases the weight. Next, try to separate the lower portion of the back, and the gluteals, from the supporting surface and bring your knees to your chest.

▬ Easier variation

The incline and added weight held by your legs makes the difficulty of the principal exercise a given. In order to reduce intensity, you can do the same movement but eliminate the weight between your legs. You can also lessen the inclination of the support in order to further reduce the difficulty of the exercise. Remember to separate your gluteals from the bench and move your knees toward your chest.

STARTING POSITION

Technical considerations

■ Eliminate the movement of the hips and knees and focus on flexing your trunk.

■ You must separate the lower portion of your back from the support.

■ Hold yourself to the upper portion of the support with your hands so that you do not slide, particularly on inclining surfaces.

FINAL POSITION

Harder variation ✚

If adding an incline to the elevation of the hips increases the difficulty of the exercise, this difficulty will be even greater if you reach the maximum incline, which is the vertical position. To do this, hang from a fixed element by both hands and perform the same trunk flex so that your thighs are raised.

34 Crunches With Weight and Extended Arms

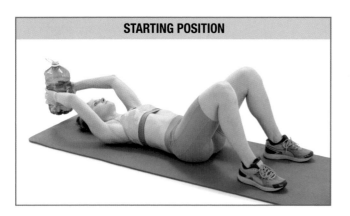

STARTING POSITION

The crunch is a classic movement for the muscular development of the abdominals. There is a myth that states that adding weight to abdominal exercises is harmful and can deform the abdomen. However, nothing could be further from reality since adding intensity to the exercise helps to boost muscular hypertrophy so this muscle is not absolutely distinct. As long as you are careful with technique and adapt the resistance to your level of development and experience, you should not experience any issues.

+

8

MUSCULAR INTENSITY

−

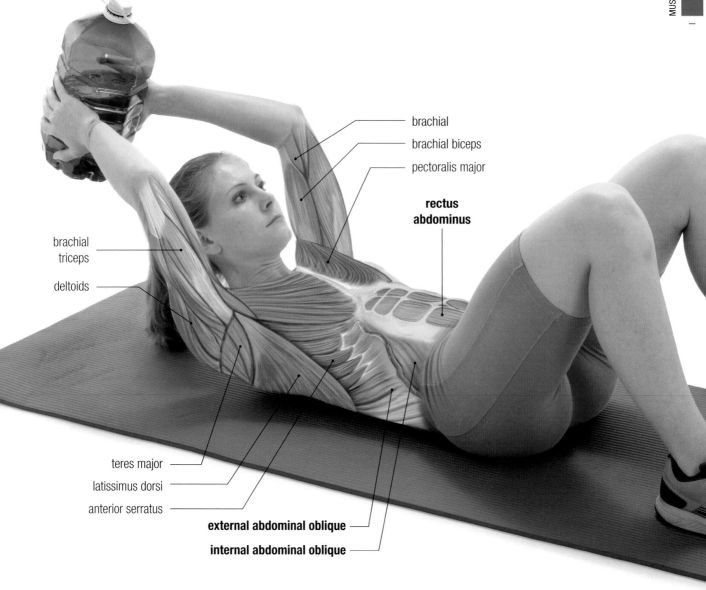

brachial

brachial biceps

pectoralis major

rectus abdominus

brachial triceps

deltoids

teres major

latissimus dorsi

anterior serratus

external abdominal oblique

internal abdominal oblique

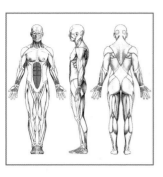

Execution

Lie facing up with the palms of your hands on the floor. Use a mat or a soft surface, since working directly on the ground is not advisable. Hold a somewhat heavy item with both hands and locate it above your head. Contract your abdominal muscles until the upper part of the back is separated from the floor by a few centimeters.

Technical considerations

■ Your shoulders and elbows must remain motionless during the execution of the exercise.

■ Limit the movement to flexing your trunk.

■ Remember that the move-ment must be very short, and barely perceptible.

▬ Easier variation

You can decrease the difficulty doing exactly the same exercise, but without holding any load. The simple act of extending your arms will already increase the resistance a little, due to the movement of the center of gravity. This step will make the exercise harder to perform than the classic crunch, but less difficult than the crunch of the principal exercise.

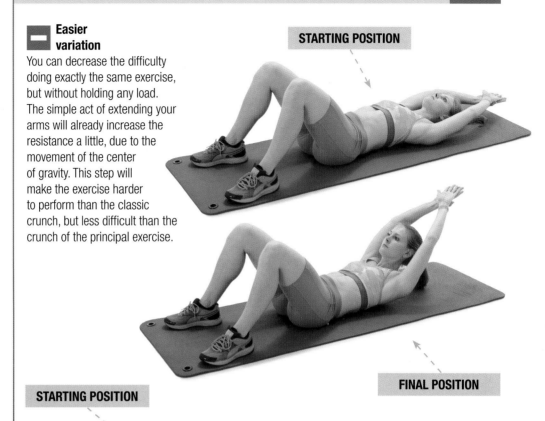

STARTING POSITION

FINAL POSITION

STARTING POSITION

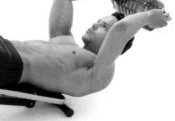

FINAL POSITION

Harder variation ✚

In order to increase intensity and make this variation a very hard alternative, it is enough to add a second factor which will contribute difficulty to the principal exercise (in addition to the weight) to work the abdominals. This factor is inclination. In this case, given that the weight is in your hands, it will be the shoulders that must remain below the hips.

35 Suspension Inverted Crunch

Although up until now we have shown the use of nylon belts in suspension with your hands, it is also possible to hold them with your feet and support your hands on the floor. Working this way will make it possible to perform various, difficult and effective exercises for your abdominal muscles.

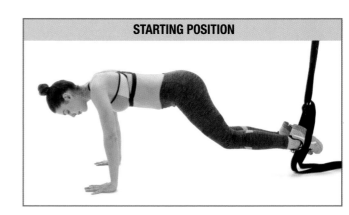

STARTING POSITION

Execution

Put the belt around a raised support and tie a knot with the ends to make loops. Place yourself on all fours and put a foot through each loop. Separate your knees, but keep your hands supported on the floor and your feet in the loops. Flex your trunk, minimizing the movement of your hips so that your feet move a few centimeters closer to your hands.

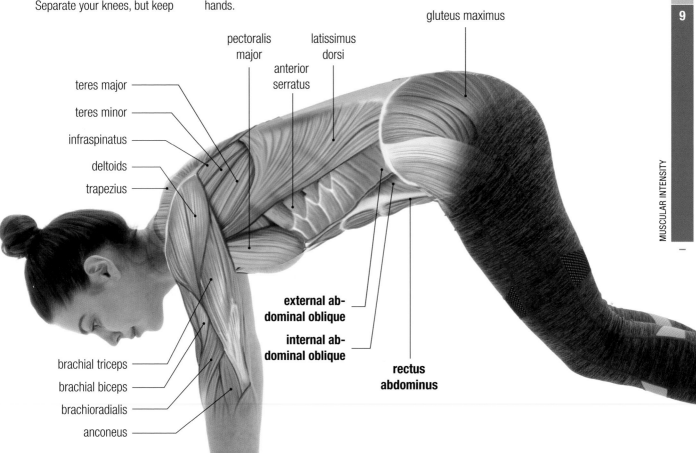

teres major

teres minor

infraspinatus

deltoids

trapezius

pectoralis major

anterior serratus

latissimus dorsi

gluteus maximus

brachial triceps

brachial biceps

brachioradialis

anconeus

external abdominal oblique

internal abdominal oblique

rectus abdominus

MUSCULAR INTENSITY

+

9

−

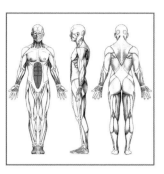

Technical considerations

- Minimize the movement to flex your trunk.

- Arch your back upward and never toward the ground.

- Your suspended feet should be close to the floor, without touching it.

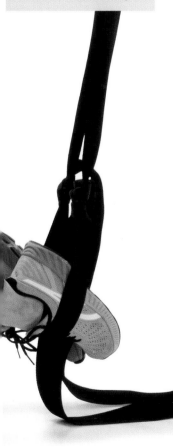

➖ Easier variation

There is a somewhat simpler variation which requires little preparation. It consists of getting down on all fours, supported by your hands and toes. In order to promote the sliding of your toes on the floor, wear socks, or put a rag under your sneakers. Contract the abdominals and flex your trunk, drawing your hands and feet toward each other.

➕ Harder variation

In order to increase the level of difficulty, beginning with the starting position of the principal exercise, flex and rotate your trunk, using more than half of your oblique abdominal muscles. This time, your knees should move from side to side, which involves these being flexed along with your hips, going from the starting position, in which these joints are extended.

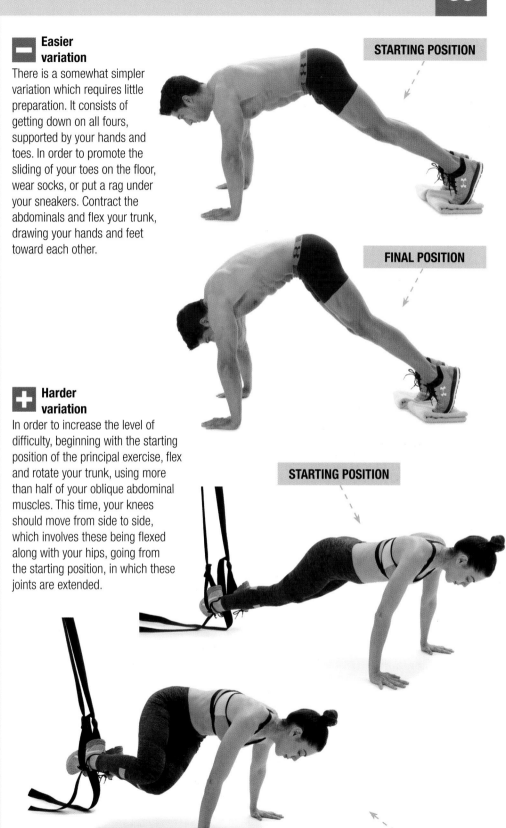

STARTING POSITION

FINAL POSITION

STARTING POSITION

FINAL POSITION

36 | Side Plank

The side plank is an exercise that does not require any type of equipment and works the oblique muscles of the abdomen. In general, the final position is reached and held for several seconds, thus executing an isometric contraction. However, as in the rest of the exercises, it can also be done isometrically, with the usual repetitions of the movement.

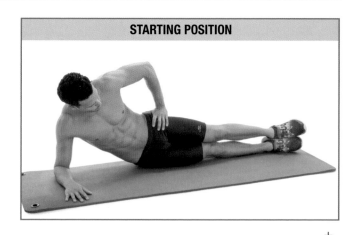

STARTING POSITION

Execution

Lie on your side, directly on the floor, or on a mat. Keep your foot, thigh and forearm in contact with the floor as support. From here, try to align the the trunk with the lower extremities so that only one foot and one forearm remain in contact with the floor. As you do this, your hip will progressively separate from the floor.

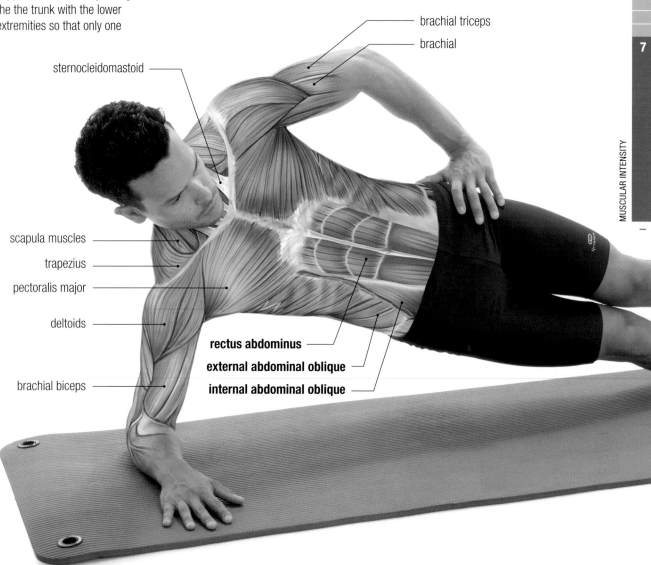

brachial triceps

brachial

sternocleidomastoid

scapula muscles

trapezius

pectoralis major

deltoids

rectus abdominus

external abdominal oblique

internal abdominal oblique

brachial biceps

MUSCULAR INTENSITY

+

7

−

ALTERNATIVE EXERCISES

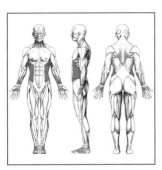

Technical considerations

■ Try to find a stable support.

■ You can put one foot in front of the other if this is helpful to you in achieving stability.

■ If you feel too much pain at any support point, use a mat, a cushion or any other item that will alleviate pressure from that area.

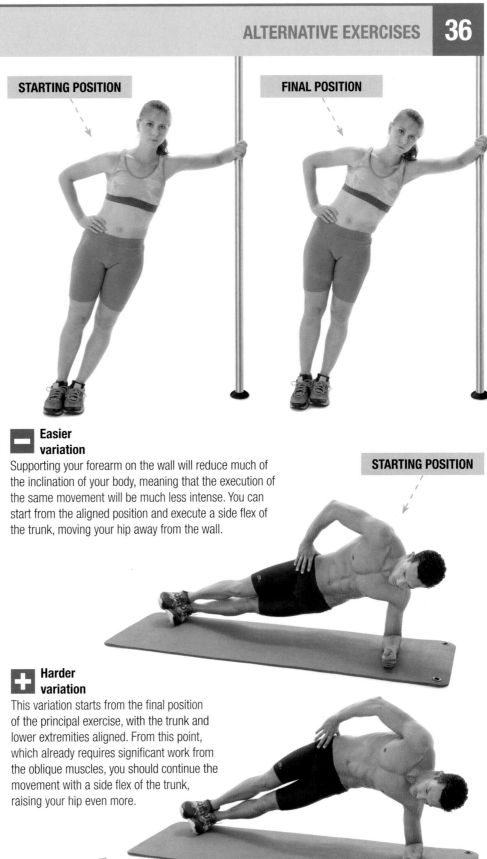

STARTING POSITION

FINAL POSITION

STARTING POSITION

FINAL POSITION

— Easier variation

Supporting your forearm on the wall will reduce much of the inclination of your body, meaning that the execution of the same movement will be much less intense. You can start from the aligned position and execute a side flex of the trunk, moving your hip away from the wall.

+ Harder variation

This variation starts from the final position of the principal exercise, with the trunk and lower extremities aligned. From this point, which already requires significant work from the oblique muscles, you should continue the movement with a side flex of the trunk, raising your hip even more.

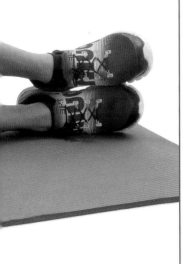

37 | Side Crunch

The abdominal obliques, very often forgotten due to their reduced influence on general physical appearance, are an important muscle group for enjoying adequate body balance and function. Nonetheless, a side crunch that is well-executed often requires a point at which to fix your feet.

Execution

Lie down on your side on a mat or other surface, preferably cushioned. Whenever you can, fix your feet or ask a training partner to hold them to the floor, one in front of the other. Put your hands behind your neck without pulling on your head, and flex your trunk sideways until your side separates from the floor.

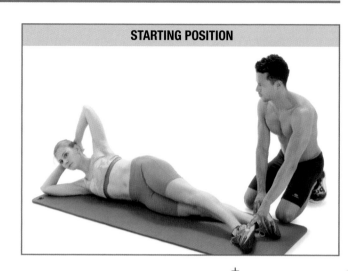

STARTING POSITION

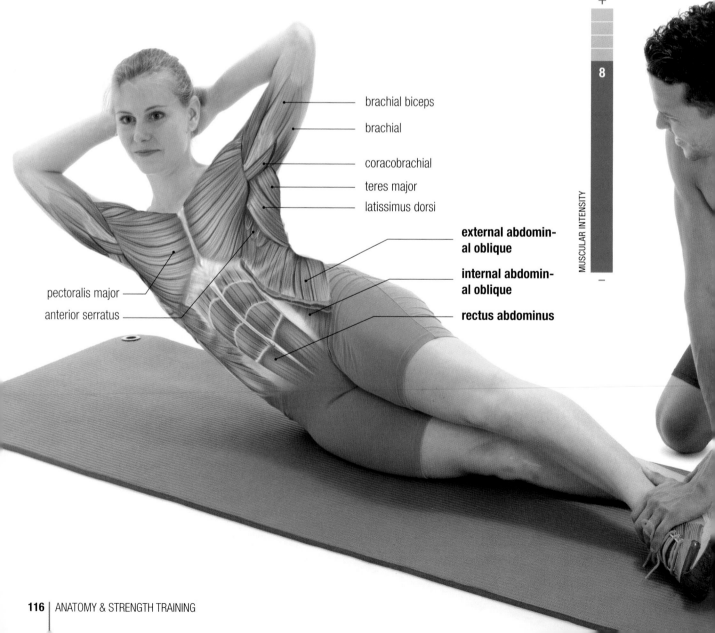

brachial biceps

brachial

coracobrachial

teres major

latissimus dorsi

external abdominal oblique

internal abdominal oblique

rectus abdominus

pectoralis major

anterior serratus

MUSCULAR INTENSITY

+

8

−

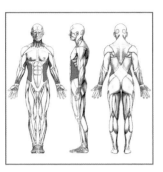

Technical considerations

- Place one foot in front of the other so that both feet are on the floor.

- It is a good idea to set your feet so that they remain motionless, or to ask a training partner to hold them.

- It is a good idea to place something between the floor and your body, such as a mat.

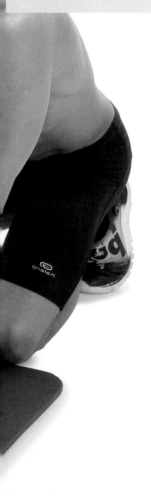

➖ Easier variation

The abdominal obliques can be worked with less intensity starting from a standing position. To do this, hold a heavy object in one hand and execute successive side flexes of the trunk toward the side opposite the load, causing the load to rise and fall a few centimeters with each repetition.

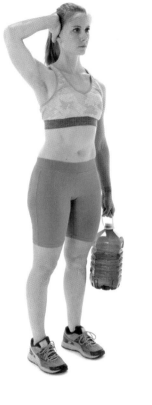

STARTING POSITION

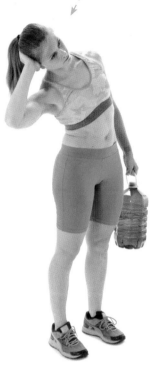

FINAL POSITION

➕ Harder variation

This variation is technically more demanding. The starting position is the same as that of the principal exercise, but here, your feet are not held down, and when you execute the side flex of the trunk, both your feet and the upper portion of the trunk separate from the floor.

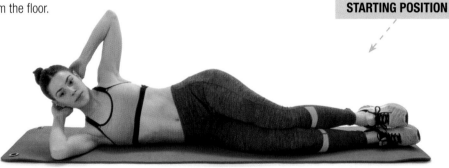

STARTING POSITION

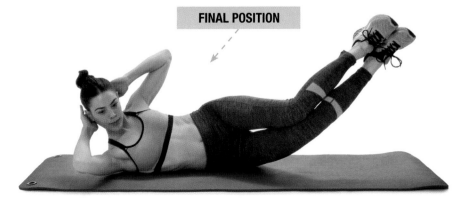

FINAL POSITION

38 | Hip Raises With Weight

The gluteus maximus is a muscle that, if worked properly, contributes a great deal to the general aesthetic of the body, since it controls the silhouette. Traditionally, women have been more concerned with this area of the body than men, but this is changing, since more and more men are aware that they cannot achieve balance if they neglect areas in their training sessions.

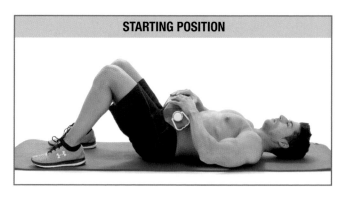

STARTING POSITION

Execution

Lie face-up with your hips and knees flexed so that the soles of your feet are supported on the floor. Place a weight on your hips and hold it with both hands. Contract your glutes so that your hips extend and lift the weight. At the highest point, the trunk and thighs will be aligned and the body will be supported on the upper portion of the back.

+

5

MUSCULAR INTENSITY

−

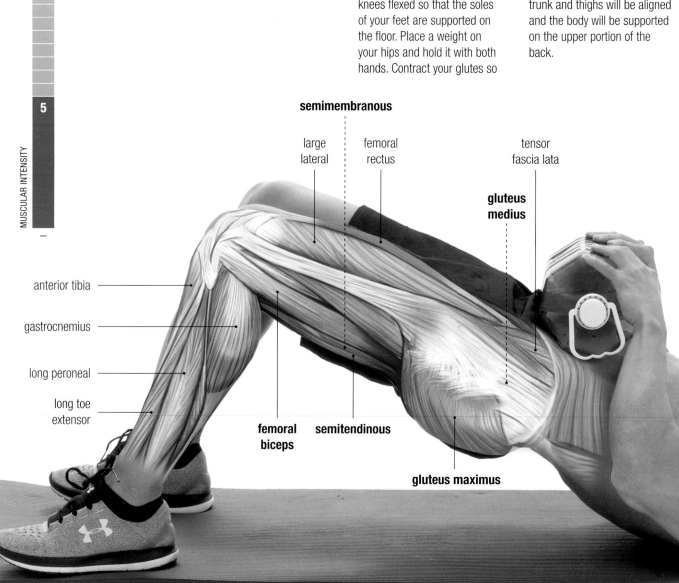

semimembranous

large lateral

femoral rectus

tensor fascia lata

gluteus medius

anterior tibia

gastrocnemius

long peroneal

long toe extensor

femoral biceps

semitendinous

gluteus maximus

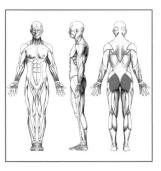

Technical considerations

■ Hold the weight with each hand.

■ Keep your neck relaxed.

➖ Easier variation

The principal exercise is not highly demanding so if you are a beginner, this variation, without added weight, will be even more accessible to you. Place your hands at your sides and, lying on the floor, execute the same movement as in the principal version.

STARTING POSITION

FINAL POSITION

➕ Harder variation

One way to increase the resistance when it is not possible to keep adding an external weight, such as when you have specialized equipment, is to execute the exercise unilaterally. To do this, lift one leg and leave all of the work to the other leg, and then change legs after a few repetitions.

STARTING POSITION

FINAL POSITION

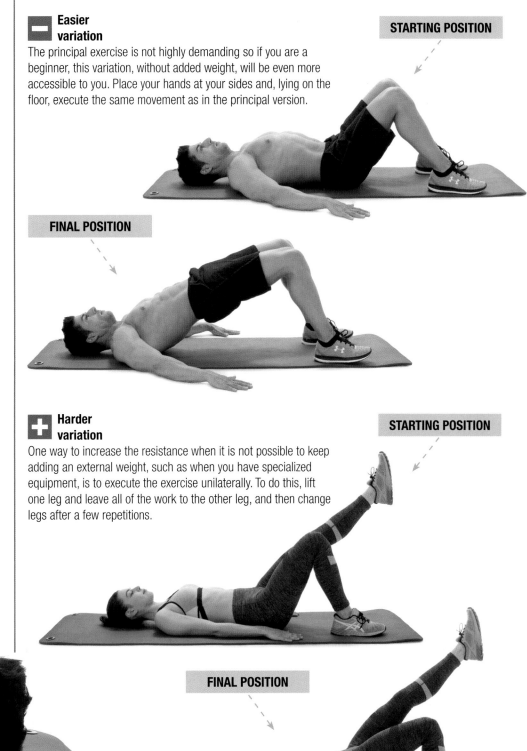

39 | **Double Kick**

The hip extension movement is a determining element in working the gluteus maximus, and the kick is one of the basic exercises to execute. For this purpose, the double kick will make it possible to work both sides of the glutes simultaneously in an effective and time-efficient manner.

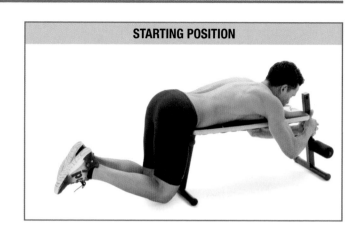

STARTING POSITION

Execution

Place the upper half of your body on a bench or similar surface so that your hips and knees are flexed and your lower extremities are not on the bench. Grasp the support firmly with both hands.

Extend the hips and knees progressively so that the lower extremities are raised and aligned with your trunk, finishing in a slightly arched body position.

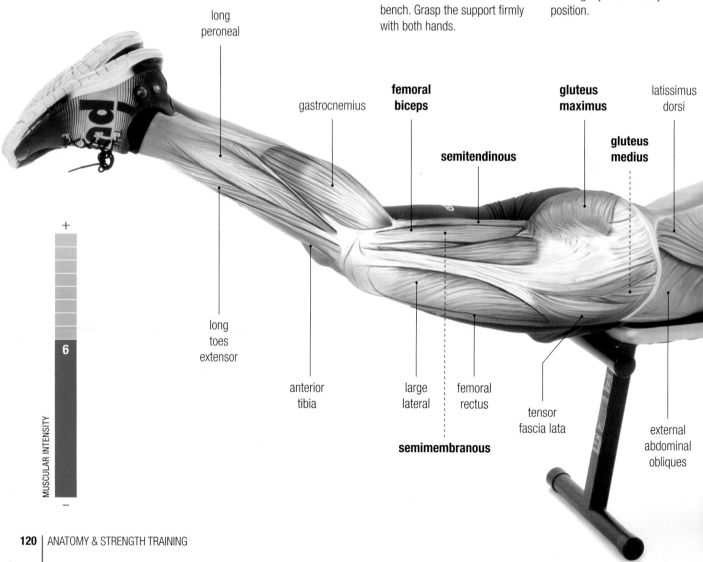

long peroneal

gastrocnemius

femoral biceps

gluteus maximus

latissimus dorsi

semitendinous

gluteus medius

long toes extensor

anterior tibia

large lateral

femoral rectus

tensor fascia lata

external abdominal obliques

semimembranous

MUSCULAR INTENSITY

+

6

−

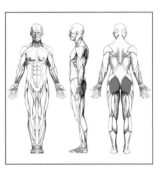

Technical considerations

■ Use an element that is stable enough to serve as a support.

■ You can reduce the intensity a bit by keeping your knees flexed throughout the exercise.

■ Extend your hips as far as you can.

▬ Easier variation

In order to execute this exercise, you can begin from an all-fours position without using any support element. To complete the exercise, you should execute the movement for each hip separately, completing a series for each glute. The intensity of each series will be less, although you will obtain just as effective results.

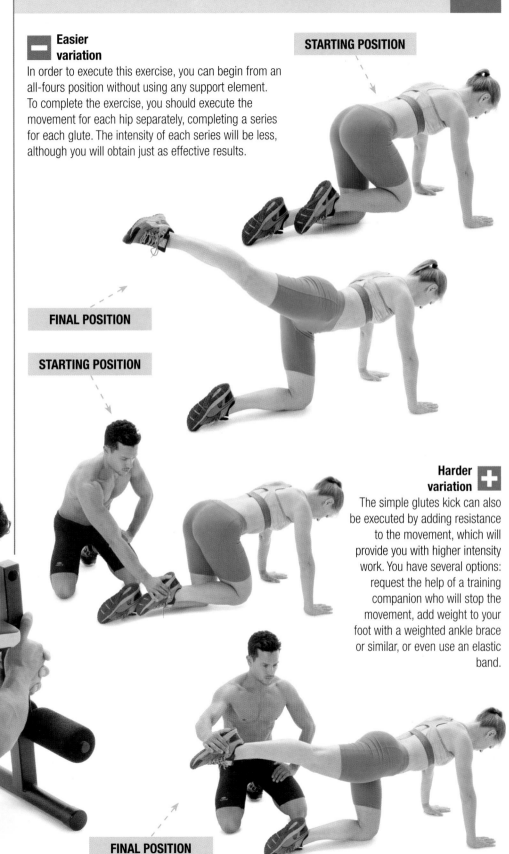

STARTING POSITION

FINAL POSITION

STARTING POSITION

Harder variation ✚

The simple glutes kick can also be executed by adding resistance to the movement, which will provide you with higher intensity work. You have several options: request the help of a training companion who will stop the movement, add weight to your foot with a weighted ankle brace or similar, or even use an elastic band.

FINAL POSITION

40 Resistance Kicks

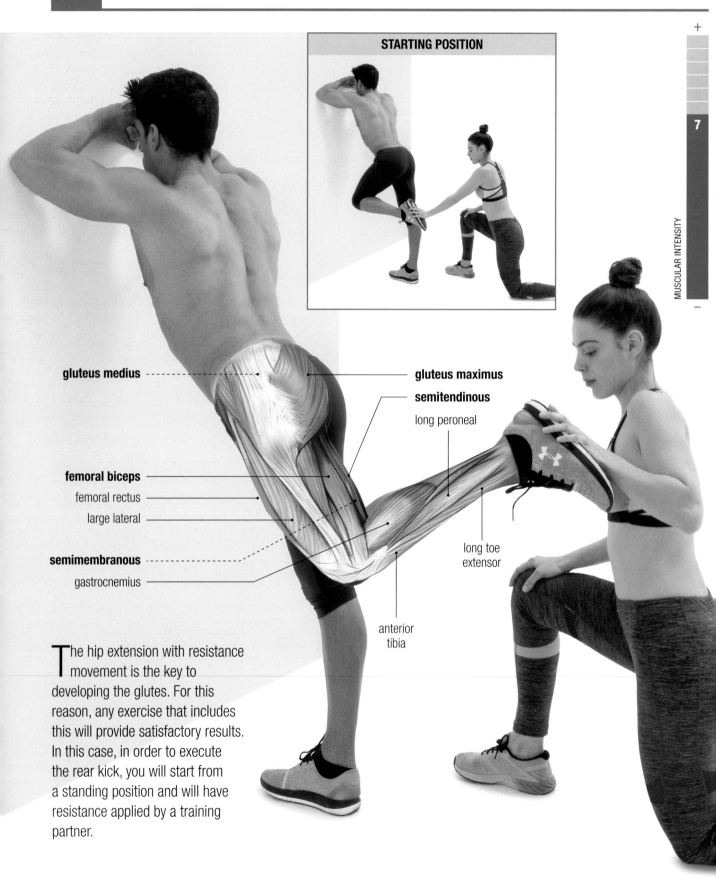

STARTING POSITION

MUSCULAR INTENSITY

+

7

−

gluteus medius

gluteus maximus

semitendinous

long peroneal

femoral biceps

femoral rectus

large lateral

long toe extensor

semimembranous

gastrocnemius

anterior tibia

The hip extension with resistance movement is the key to developing the glutes. For this reason, any exercise that includes this will provide satisfactory results. In this case, in order to execute the rear kick, you will start from a standing position and will have resistance applied by a training partner.

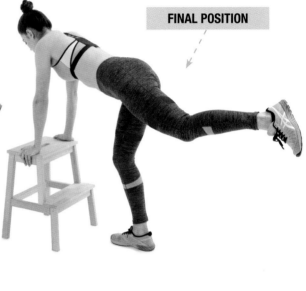

STARTING POSITION

Easier variation ▬

If you prefer to execute the kicking movement without the help of a partner, you will need to find a stable stool or chair on which to support your hands. Incline your trunk forward and then extend and flex the hip you are working, several times. Then, repeat the process with the opposite extremity.

FINAL POSITION

Execution

Stand in front of a wall, railing or post, with your trunk slightly inclined toward it. You can support yourself with your hands or forearms. Have one foot curled up like a flamenco while your partner pushes on the sole of the foot. Contract your glute, extend the hip and push your training partner's hand, while your partner provides adequate resistance.

➕ Harder variation

If you wish to train alone, but you need the added resistance of a heavy element, you can use a loaded bag, or a weighted ankle brace. If you choose the bag, you should execute the exercise on a step ladder or similar so that the bag does not hit the floor with each repetition.

Technical considerations

- Support your hands or forearms on a firm surface so that you do not lose your balance when pushing.

- Execute the kicking movement slowly.

- Start from the position with the hip flexed in order to extend the posterior movement.

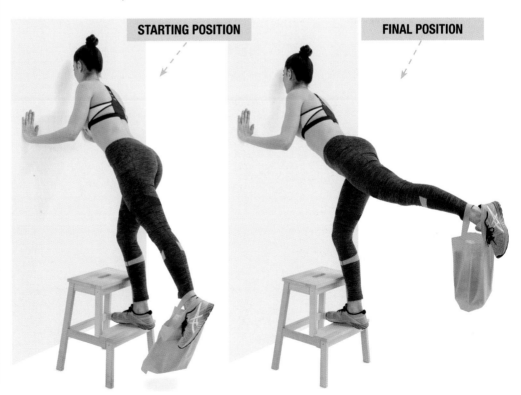

STARTING POSITION

FINAL POSITION

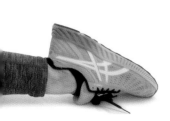

41 Squats With Weights

Squats are the first exercise that usually come to mind when we talk about training legs. Nonetheless, this classic strength exercise does not only provide excellent results for the thigh muscles, but also strengthens the glutes and erector muscles in the spine, among others.

STARTING POSITION

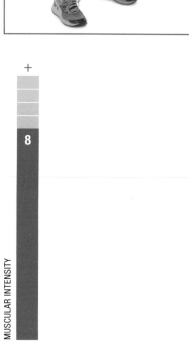

MUSCULAR INTENSITY

+

8

−

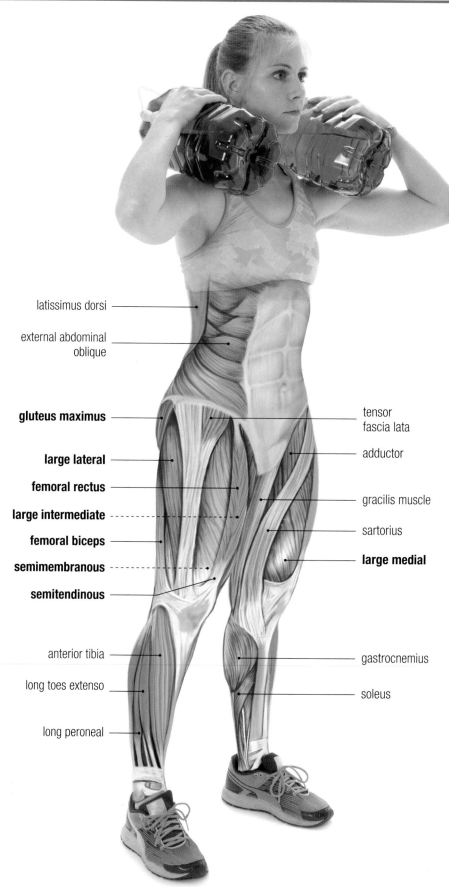

latissimus dorsi

external abdominal oblique

gluteus maximus

large lateral

femoral rectus

large intermediate

femoral biceps

semimembranous

semitendinous

anterior tibia

long toes extenso

long peroneal

tensor fascia lata

adductor

gracilis muscle

sartorius

large medial

gastrocnemius

soleus

Squats with weights

ALTERNATIVE EXERCISES 41

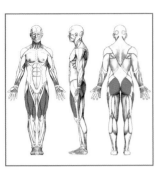

Execution

Beginning from a standing position, hold a pair of weights over your shoulders. The reason for using the already classic water jugs is their versatility and the ability to regulate their weight, but you can also use another heavy object.
Flex your knees and hips to 90 degrees, or even lower. Then extend them again, lifting the weight, until you return to the starting position.

Technical considerations

- Reaching a very low point in your descent can damage your knees.

- Avoid locking your extended legs when you reach the highest point.

- Keep your spine extended when you reach the highest point.

➖ Easier variation

The same exercise performed without weights will be a good option for beginners or those who are out of shape. Extend your arms forward to improve your stability and balance during the execution of the squat.

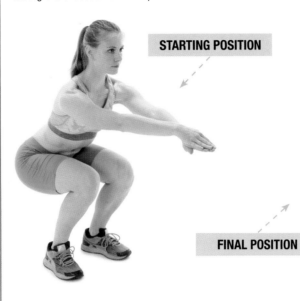
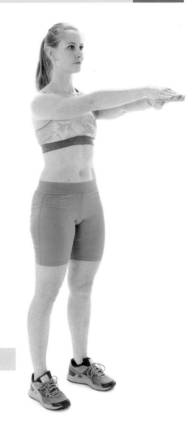

STARTING POSITION

FINAL POSITION

➕ Harder variation

Regardless of how it may seem, executing the same squat without a weight and only one leg is an almost impossible movement for the majority of people, particularly those who wish to attain the 90-degree knee and hip position, or go even further. This variant of higher intensity is within the reach of very few athletes.

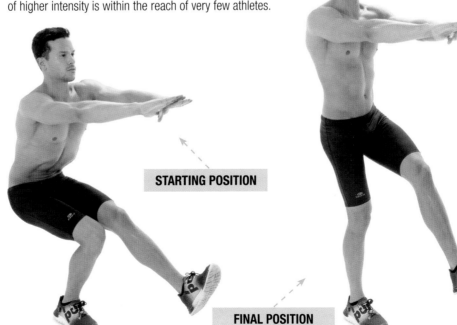

STARTING POSITION

FINAL POSITION

42 Suspension Squats

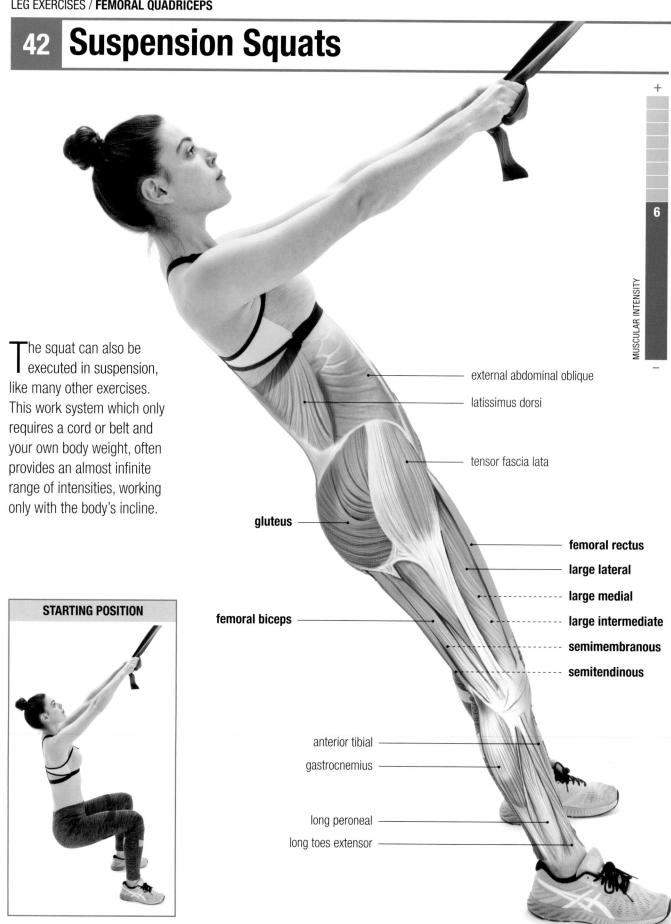

The squat can also be executed in suspension, like many other exercises. This work system which only requires a cord or belt and your own body weight, often provides an almost infinite range of intensities, working only with the body's incline.

MUSCULAR INTENSITY

+

6

−

external abdominal oblique

latissimus dorsi

tensor fascia lata

gluteus

femoral rectus

large lateral

large medial

large intermediate

femoral biceps

semimembranous

semitendinous

STARTING POSITION

anterior tibial

gastrocnemius

long peroneal

long toes extensor

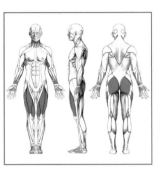

Execution

Pass the nylon belt through an elevated support and hold one end with each hand. Hang, leaning backward a little until your knees and elbows are extended and your arms are in front of you.

Flex your knees and hips, lowering your center of gravity and then extend them, lifting your own weight until you return to the standing position.

Technical considerations

- If you have pain or problems with your knees, try not to flex them more than 90 degrees.

- Keep your back straight.

- Do not flex your elbows or tense your arms during the movement.

➖ Easier variation

This variation slightly reduces the difficulty and requires less preparation. You only need to support your back against the wall, keeping your feet slightly forward. Flex your knees and hips, allowing your back to slide downward along the wall. Hold the position for a few seconds at the lowest point and then stand up again.

➕ Harder variation

One way to increase the intensity of an exercise without increasing resistance from the outside is to execute it unilaterally. In this case, from the final position of the principal exercise, raise one foot and perform the same exercise, lifting the weight with only one extremity; this way, an exercise of average difficulty becomes another one that is very difficult.

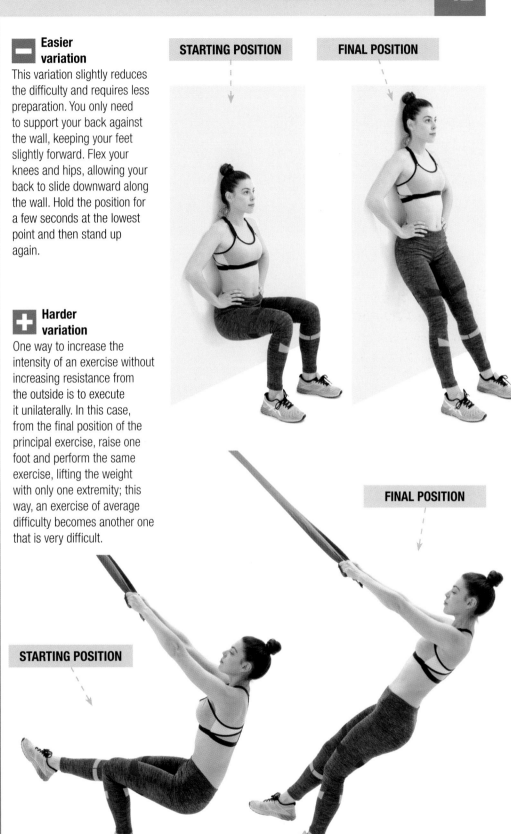

STARTING POSITION

FINAL POSITION

FINAL POSITION

STARTING POSITION

43 | Lunges With Weights

Without a doubt, lunges, along with squats and leg press exercises, are the 3 top quadriceps exercises. In addition, they can be executed in different ways, one of them being by using weights to increase their difficulty. This is an essential exercise which must be included in your legs routine.

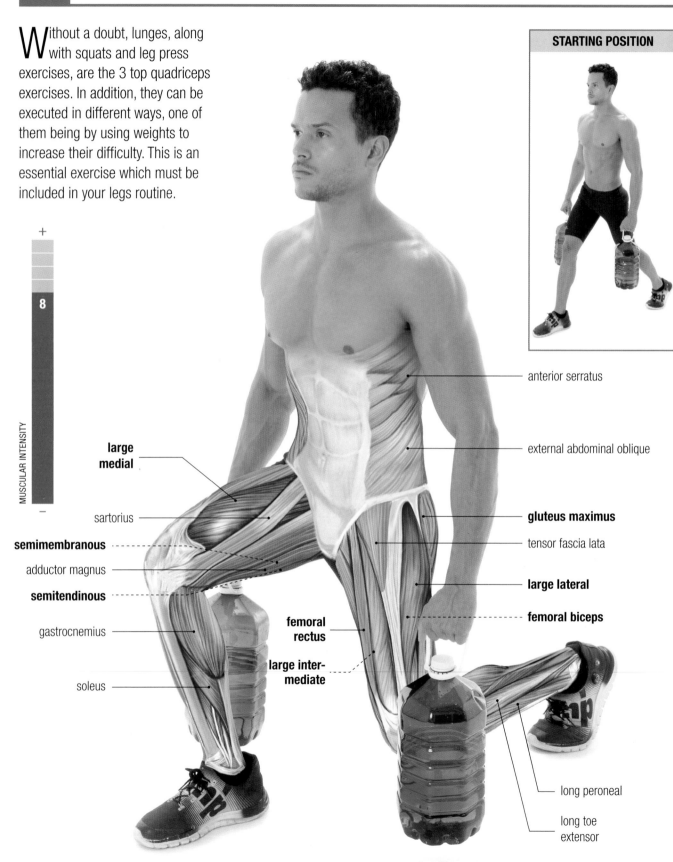

STARTING POSITION

MUSCULAR INTENSITY

+

8

−

anterior serratus

external abdominal oblique

large medial

sartorius

semimembranous

adductor magnus

semitendinous

gastrocnemius

femoral rectus

large inter- mediate

soleus

gluteus maximus

tensor fascia lata

large lateral

femoral biceps

long peroneal

long toe extensor

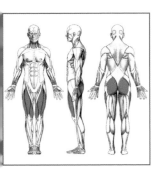

Execution

Place one foot in front of the other and hold a weight in each hand. You can substitute the customary water jugs with any other item, including with a single item to be held by both hands. Flex your knees while lowering your center of gravity. At the lowest point of the movement, both knees should be flexed to 90 degrees but without the knee in back touching the floor.

Technical considerations

■ When you reach the lowest point, try not to hit the floor with your knee.

■ Begin at a balanced position and perform the exercise slowly.

■ Try not to flex your knees more than 90 degrees.

▬ Easier variation

The same exercise can be performed without weights, making its execution easier. The movement is exactly the same, but executing it without weight is an advantage for beginning athletes, for example those who have difficulties maintaining balance or who are still learning the technique.

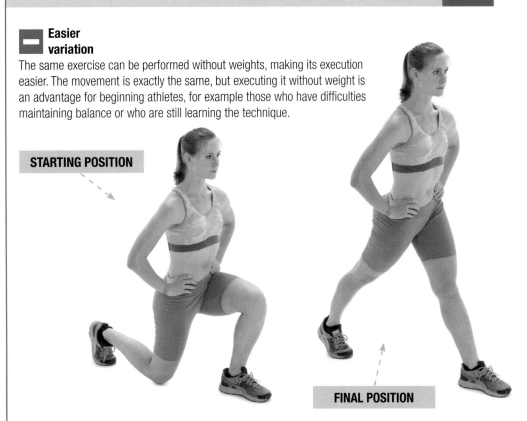

STARTING POSITION

FINAL POSITION

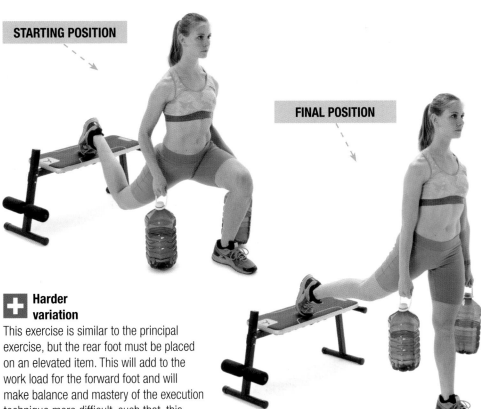

STARTING POSITION

FINAL POSITION

✚ Harder variation

This exercise is similar to the principal exercise, but the rear foot must be placed on an elevated item. This will add to the work load for the forward foot and will make balance and mastery of the execution technique more difficult, such that, this variant of the lunge with weight will become more challenging.

44 Reverse Incline

It is always preferable to work with the broadest possible ranges of movement, however, since a variety of exercises must prevail in routines, you will have to include exercises in them that may have incomplete ranges of motion. This should not be a taboo, and you should not think of it as something negative, but rather as a way to enrich your repertory of exercises.

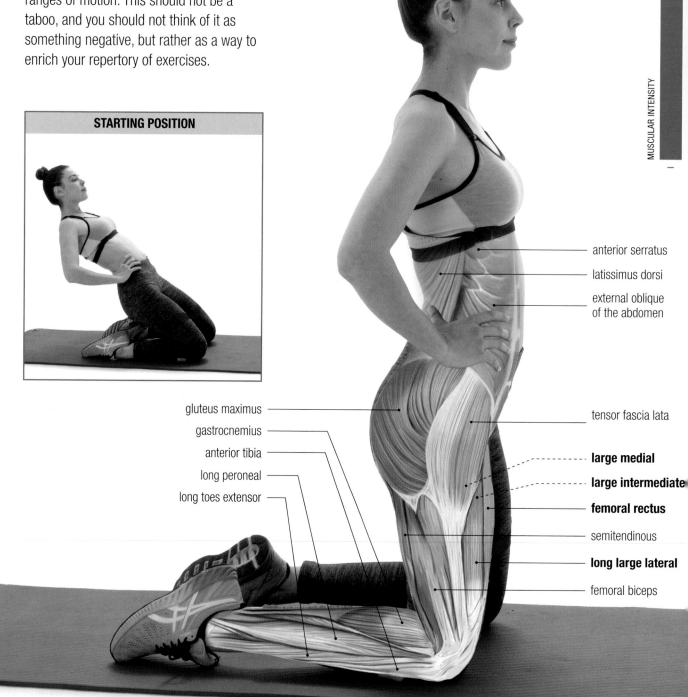

STARTING POSITION

MUSCULAR INTENSITY

8

anterior serratus

latissimus dorsi

external oblique
of the abdomen

tensor fascia lata

large medial

large intermediate

femoral rectus

semitendinous

long large lateral

femoral biceps

gluteus maximus

gastrocnemius

anterior tibia

long peroneal

long toes extensor

ALTERNATIVE EXERCISES 44

Execution

Kneel on a mat, or place something soft under your knees, for example a towel, in order to protect them. Align the thighs and trunk. Lean backward while the work of your quadriceps slows down your descent. Once you reach the lowest point, return to the vertical position, using only this muscle group.

Technical considerations

- Thighs and trunk must remain in alignment throughout the entire movement.

- Try to reach the greatest possible angle of inclination before returning to vertical.

- Separate your knees slightly to maintain stability while you work out.

Easier variation

Sit on a chair or high stool with your knees flexed to 90 degrees. Place a weight on top of your feet and extend your knees forward, raising the weight until your thighs and legs are aligned. As your legs grow stronger, you will be able to progressively add more weight to a backpack and continue performing the exercise.

Harder variation

Once you are able to accomplish the principal exercise with very steep degrees of inclination, you can continue to increase the difficulty by adding weights. Place the weights on your chest, behind your neck or on top of your head, if you want to reach the highest level of difficulty.

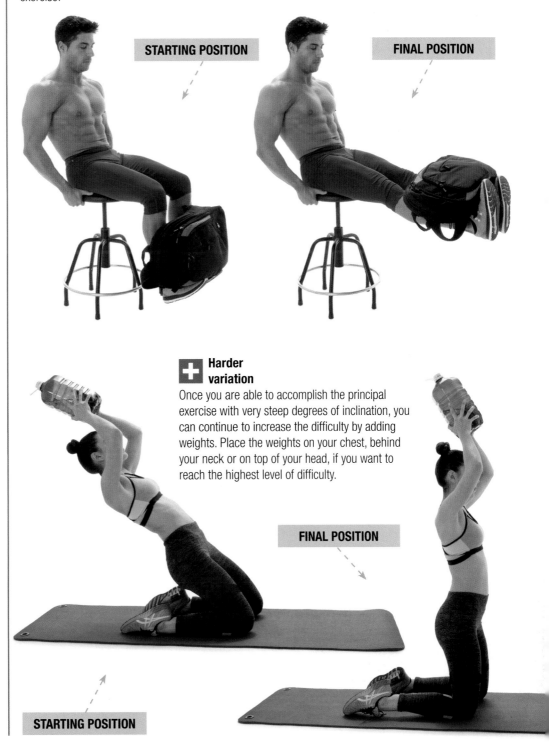

STARTING POSITION

FINAL POSITION

FINAL POSITION

STARTING POSITION

45 | Sissy Squats

The sissy squat is very popular with some people. Nonetheless, today it is not usual to see athletes working out in gyms using this exercise. Despite this, the exercise makes it possible to work the quadriceps in isolation, since it limits the participation of the glutes and hamstrings that occurs during other quadriceps exercises, such as the squat or lunges.

STARTING POSITION

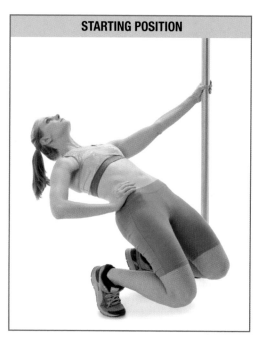

MUSCULAR INTENSITY

+

9

−

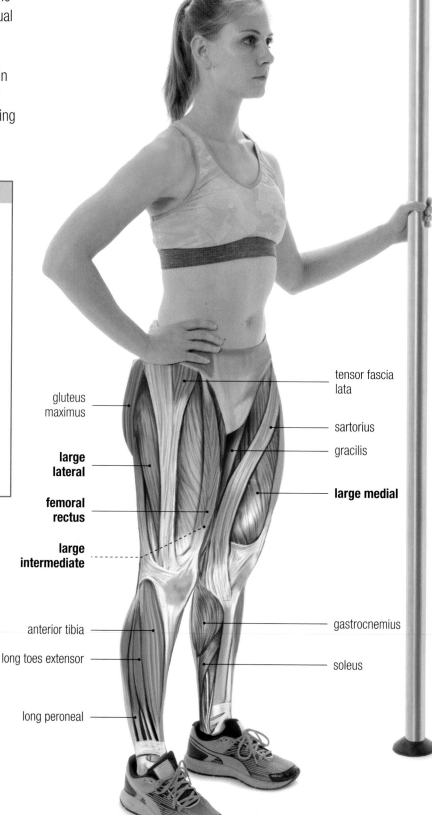

tensor fascia lata

gluteus maximus

sartorius

gracilis

large lateral

large medial

femoral rectus

large intermediate

anterior tibia

gastrocnemius

long toes extensor

soleus

long peroneal

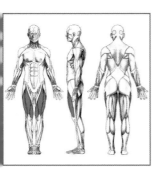

Execution

Hold on to a vertical support, whether a post, a railing, a handle or similar. Flex your knees so that your body inclines backward, with your trunk and thighs aligned. At the lowest point of the movement, support yourself on your toes so that balance is difficult to maintain. Extend your knees again, until you are standing.

Technical considerations

- Keep your thighs and trunk aligned at all times.

- Always keep one hand gripped to a support in order to maintain your balance.

▬ Easier variation

If you have a vertical support and a belt, you can do the Russian belt squat. To do this, tie together the ends of a piece of belt, place it around a support and put your legs through it so that the belt is tensed. Lower your weight and flex your knees until you are in the squat.

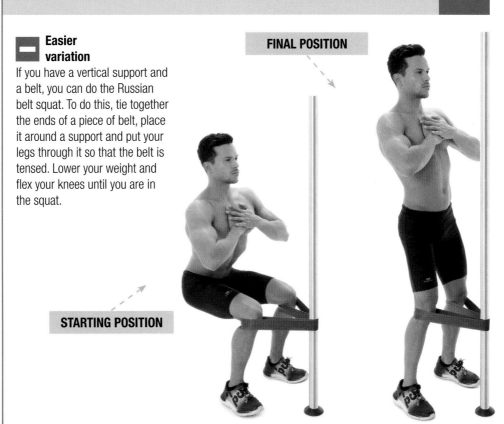

FINAL POSITION

STARTING POSITION

✚ Harder variation

The sissy squat can be executed with an added weight which you can hang from your free hand, or hold against your chest. This will add difficulty to an already difficult exercise. Do this only when you have mastered the technique and have practiced the basic variant.

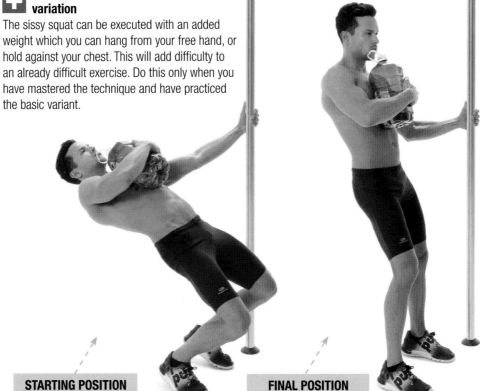

STARTING POSITION

FINAL POSITION

46 | Standing Hamstring Curl

Exercises for working the hamstrings are, without a doubt, less creative than those that are done with other muscle groups. Certainly, the development of these muscles will never be very showy, like those for the quadriceps, gastrocnemius or gluteals; nonetheless, their correct execution is essential in order to avoid imbalances which could affect your health.

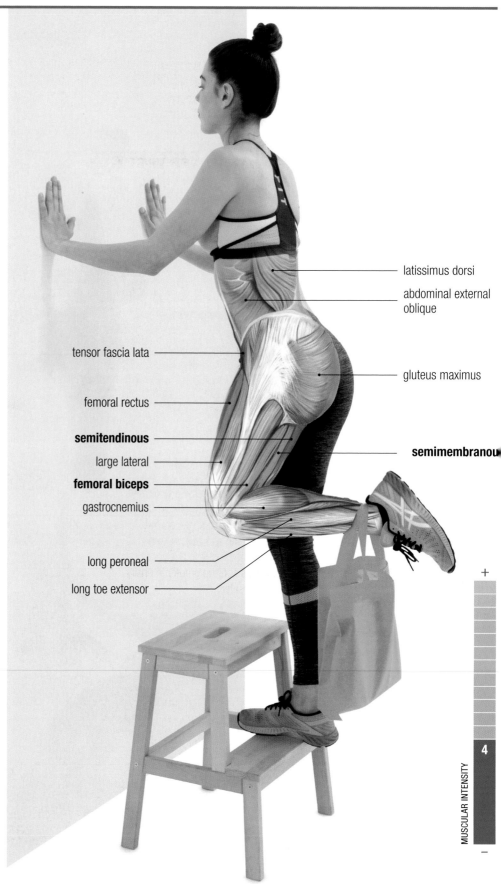

latissimus dorsi

abdominal external oblique

tensor fascia lata

gluteus maximus

femoral rectus

semitendinous

large lateral

semimembranou

femoral biceps

gastrocnemius

long peroneal

long toe extensor

MUSCULAR INTENSITY

+

4

−

STARTING POSITION

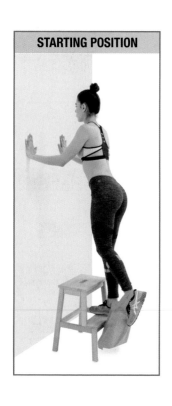

Execution

First, place a weight on your ankle. You can use a weighted ankle brace, but if you do not have one, you can use a bag filled with objects that will hang from your ankle (see the example). Support one foot on a step to prevent the bag from hitting the floor and flex and extend your knee successively to move the weight.

Technical considerations

- Try to focus the movement on your knee, keeping your hip almost motionless.

- You can support yourself with your hands or hold onto something to improve stability.

- The knee of the supporting leg must be slightly flexed.

Easier variation

If you train with a partner, you can forgo the weight and ask your partner to oppose the movement with their hand. The benefit of this variant is that the resistance can be continuously and immediately adjusted as your needs change. Don't forget that, in order to improve, the exercise must always provide a certain level of difficulty.

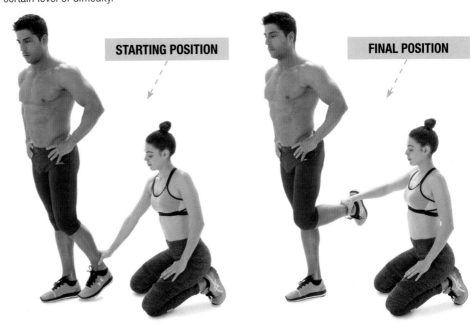

STARTING POSITION

FINAL POSITION

Harder variation

Lie facedown to lock your hip and more easily limit the movement of your knee. Ask a partner to place a belt or towel around your ankle and pull on both ends to make it difficult to flex your knee, and thus achieve greater intensity and greater results.

STARTING POSITION

FINAL POSITION

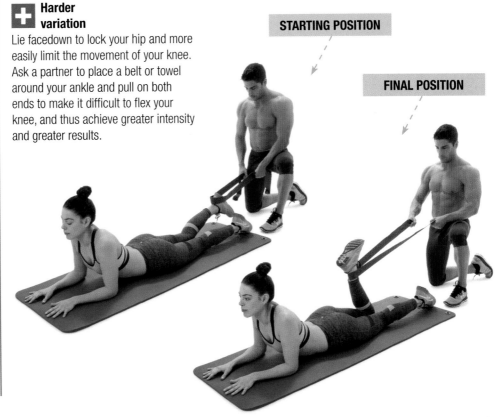

47 Romanian Deadlift

Dead weight exercises are basics for muscle development and are part of the power lifting movements, so it is common to see power athletes moving large weights when they perform this exercise. The Romanian deadlift helps to focus the work on the hamstrings and glutes.

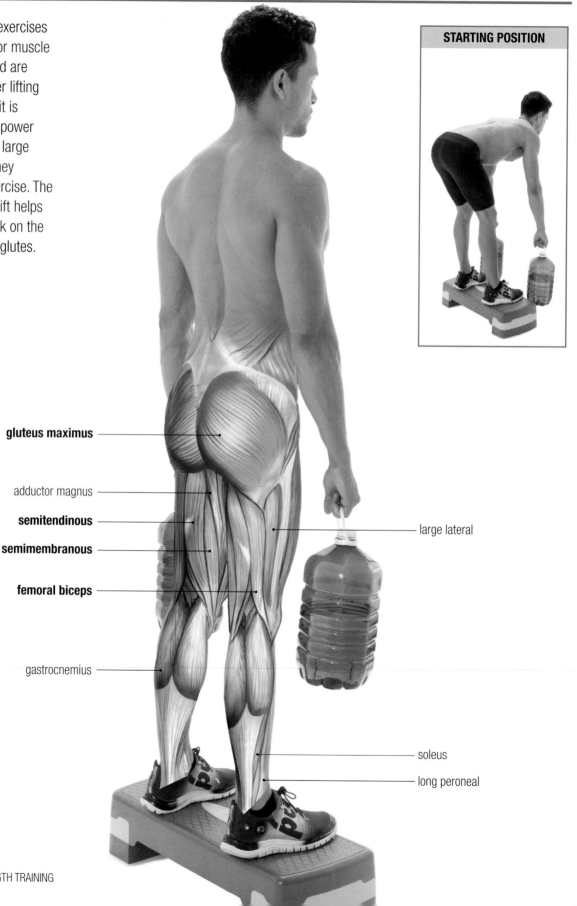

STARTING POSITION

gluteus maximus

adductor magnus

semitendinous

semimembranous

femoral biceps

gastrocnemius

large lateral

soleus

long peroneal

MUSCULAR INTENSITY

+

7

−

Execution

Hold a weight with each hand. In this case, you can use water jugs as weights. Given its range, perform the exercise on a step so that you do not lose any range of motion. Flex your hips so that your trunk leans forward while your spine remains extended. Your knees should be almost completely extended. Once you reach the end of the movement, execute the opposite movement with your hips, lifting the weight until you return to the original position.

Technical considerations

■ Your knee will remain almost completely extended throughout the movement, with minimal variation in its position.

■ Keep your back extended and the erector muscles of your spine contracted to prevent damaging your lumber spine.

▬ Easier variation

To execute a less intense variation, stand in front of a post or vertical support and have a piece of a belt with you. Tie the ends of the belt together and slip it behind the post. Put your legs through the looped ends and slide the loops up until they are just below your knees. Be sure that the belt is tensed, lean forward slowly and flex your hips so that your trunk is inclined forward. Then extend them again, until you have returned to a standing position.

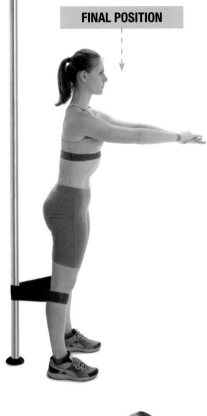

FINAL POSITION

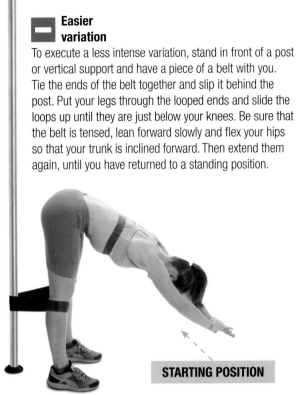

STARTING POSITION

✚ Harder variation

In order to increase the intensity of this exercise, try to execute the Romanian deadlift with one leg. The technique will be more demanding since you are starting from a less stable position. You can hold a support with one hand to improve your stability.

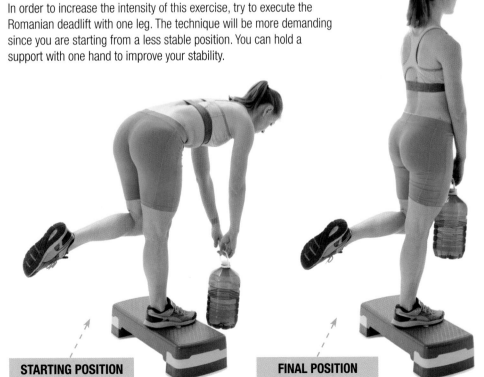

STARTING POSITION

FINAL POSITION

48 Suspension Hamstring Curls

U Once again, working in suspension will help you supplement your repertory of exercises using minimal resources. You have probably not seen this exercise before, but both its efficiency and its difficulty are remarkable and also help to strengthen the glutes, which are in isometric contraction during the exercise.

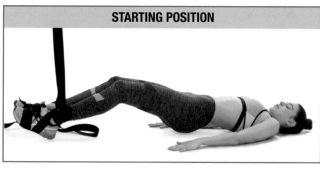

STARTING POSITION

Execution

Pass the nylon belt through an elevated support and wrap one end around each of your ankles. Lie facing up and separate your glutes from the floor, so that you are partially suspended by the ankles and with the upper portion of your back in contact with the floor. Flex your knees while you keep your trunk and thighs aligned, raising your pelvis

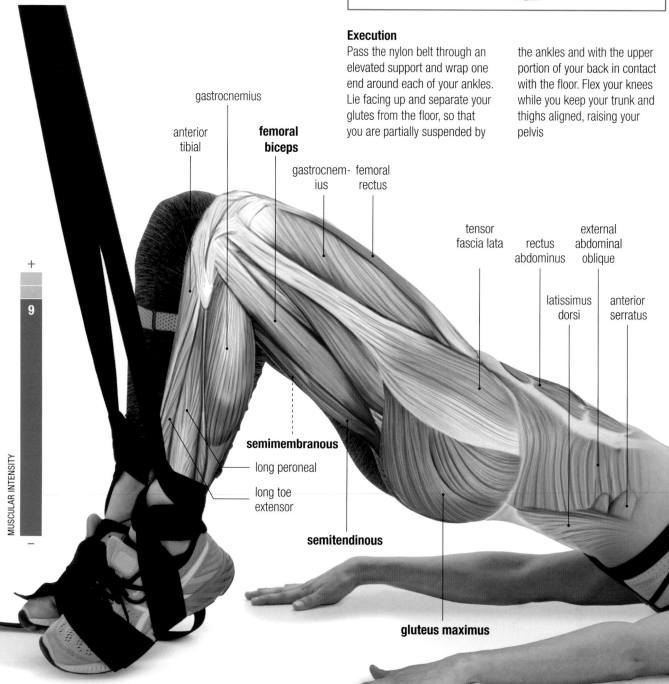

gastrocnemius

anterior tibial

femoral biceps

gastrocnem- ius

femoral rectus

tensor fascia lata

rectus abdominus

external abdominal oblique

latissimus dorsi

anterior serratus

+

9

MUSCULAR INTENSITY

−

semimembranous

long peroneal

long toe extensor

semitendinous

gluteus maximus

Suspension hamstring curls

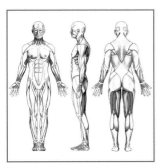

Technical considerations

■ Keep your thighs and trunk aligned throughout the movement.

■ The hip joint must remain immobile throughout the exercise.

■ The feet must be elevated a few centimeters when you begin the exercise.

— Easier variation

Given the difficulty of the principal exercise, and above all, if you are a beginner, you may be thankful for this easier alternative. Lie facedown on a mat and ask a partner to hold your ankle. Try to flex your knee while your partner applies resistance to the movement in order to make the exercise more difficult.

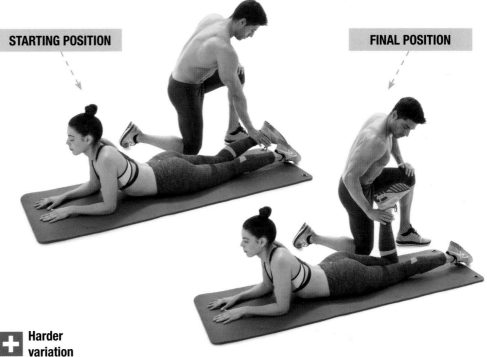

STARTING POSITION

FINAL POSITION

+ Harder variation

Kneel on a mat and fix your ankles using a fixed item, or with the assistance of a partner. Keep your trunk and thighs aligned and, progressively, allow yourself to fall forward. Once you reach the point at which you cannot continue to lower yourself without losing control, stop and return to the vertical position.

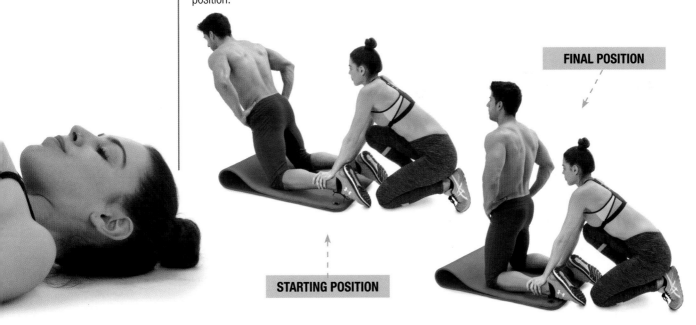

FINAL POSITION

STARTING POSITION

49 Calf Raise With Weight

The gastrocnemius (calf) muscles are often forgotten in training exercises or are inadequately worked. In part, this is due to the fact that the genetic characteristics of many athletes already provide them with a good size, with hardly any training. Even so, it must be clear that the plantar flex movement of the ankle is the most effective movement for developing them.

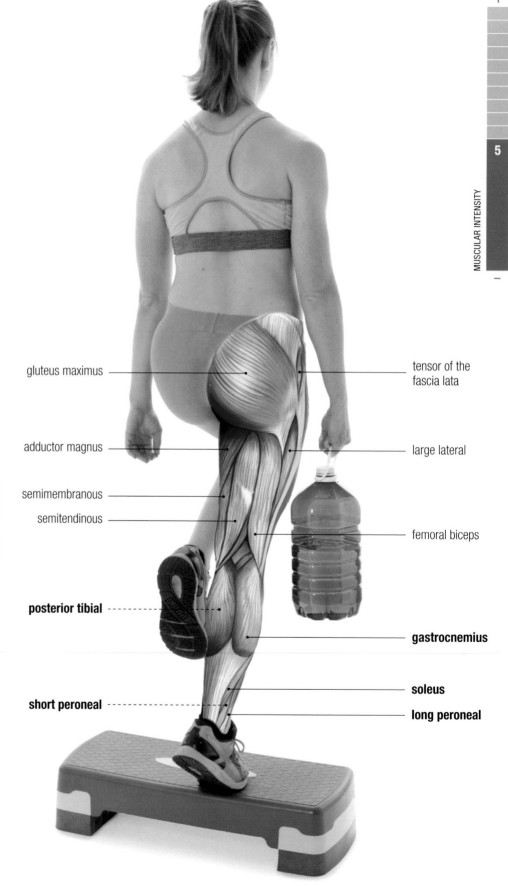

gluteus maximus

tensor of the fascia lata

adductor magnus

large lateral

semimembranous

semitendinous

femoral biceps

posterior tibial

gastrocnemius

short peroneal

soleus

long peroneal

MUSCULAR INTENSITY

+

5

−

STARTING POSITION

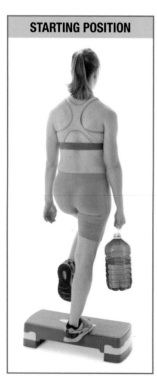

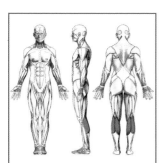

Execution

Place the toe of the only supporting foot on a step. The opposite foot must remain suspended and you should use one or both hands to hold a weighted item. At the beginning, the heel of the supporting foot should be lower than the toe. Execute a plantar ankle flex, remaining "on tiptoes" and raising your center of gravity so that your heel is located above your toe on the supporting foot.

Technical considerations

- Keep your knee extended.

- Execute the movement as broadly as possible, limiting yourself to the ankle joint.

- If you need to, support yourself with one hand.

➖ Easier variation

Executing the same exercise with the support of both feet, and without the weight will not only simplify the technique and improve your balance, but will also reduce the intensity of the muscular work. For this reason, this variation is appropriate for those who are beginners, or who have not yet mastered the technique of the exercise.

STARTING POSITION

➕ Harder variation

To do this exercise, you will need the help of a partner and a support, for example, a table or a high bench. Lean forward and put one of your forearms on the support. Ask your partner to sit on your hips (never further toward the front), because this will add significant resistance to the movement. Execute a plantar ankle flex, until you are on your toes, and then descend again.

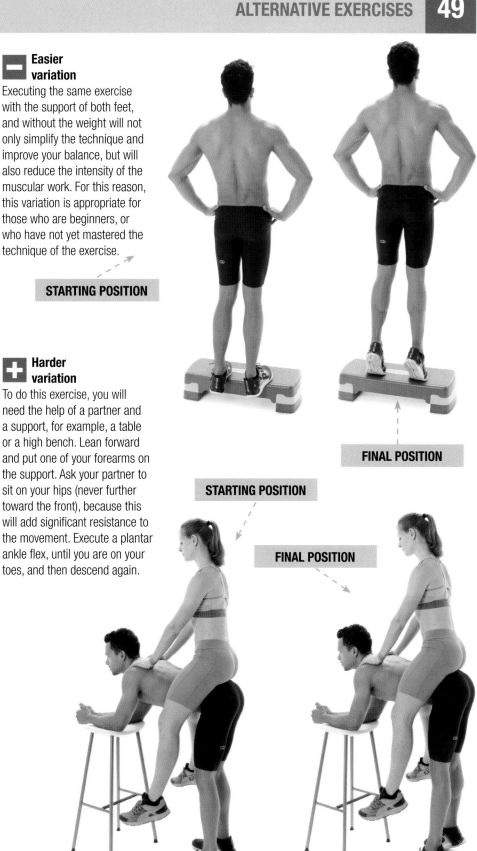

FINAL POSITION

STARTING POSITION

FINAL POSITION

50 | Suspension Calf Raise

Once more, working with a suspension trainer is great. This time, belts provide forward incline to the entire body and start from the dorsal flexing of the ankle, making it possible to execute a broad movement and, finally, effectively work the gastrocnemii and soleus.

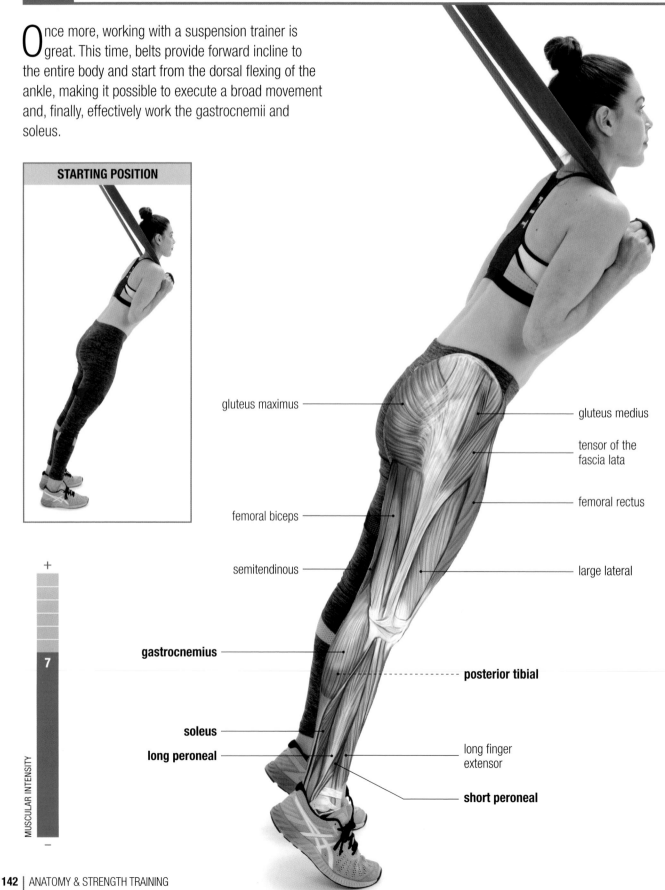

STARTING POSITION

MUSCULAR INTENSITY

+

7

−

gluteus maximus

gluteus medius

tensor of the fascia lata

femoral rectus

femoral biceps

large lateral

semitendinous

gastrocnemius

posterior tibial

soleus

long peroneal

long finger extensor

short peroneal

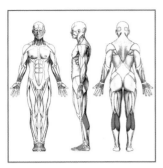

Execution

Pass the nylon belt through an elevated support and hold both ends to your shoulders, with your elbows flexed.

Lean forward, support your feet and hang from the belt. Your feet will begin at dorsal flexion and go to plantar flexion so that you end up on your toes.

Technical considerations

- Keep your knees extended throughout the movement.
- Lean forward in order to achieve a longer ankle movement.
- Keep your trunk and lower extremities aligned.

Easier variation

Stand in front of a wall and lean forward, supporting your hands on the wall. This will make it possible for you to place your ankles in a starting position of dorsal flexion, which is the best position for executing broad movements. Execute a plantar flex of both ankles, ending up on your toes. Descend and repeat the movement a number of times. Repeat the cycle several times.

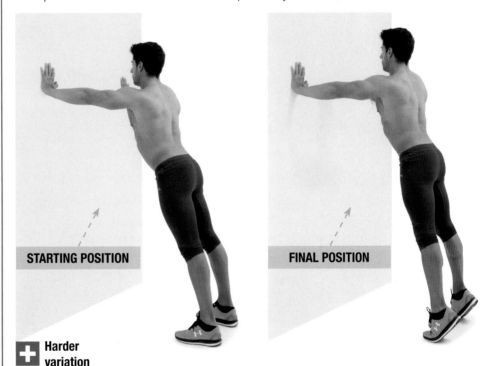

STARTING POSITION — FINAL POSITION

Harder variation

Sit on a chair or bench and ask your partner to sit on your knees. Execute a plantar ankle flexion, so that your feet finish on your toes. Remember that the knee flexion position will work the soleus muscles more than the gastrocnemii.

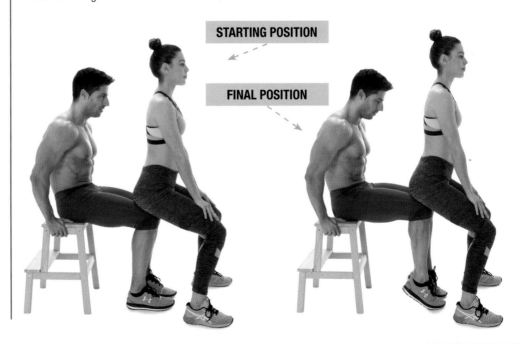

STARTING POSITION — FINAL POSITION

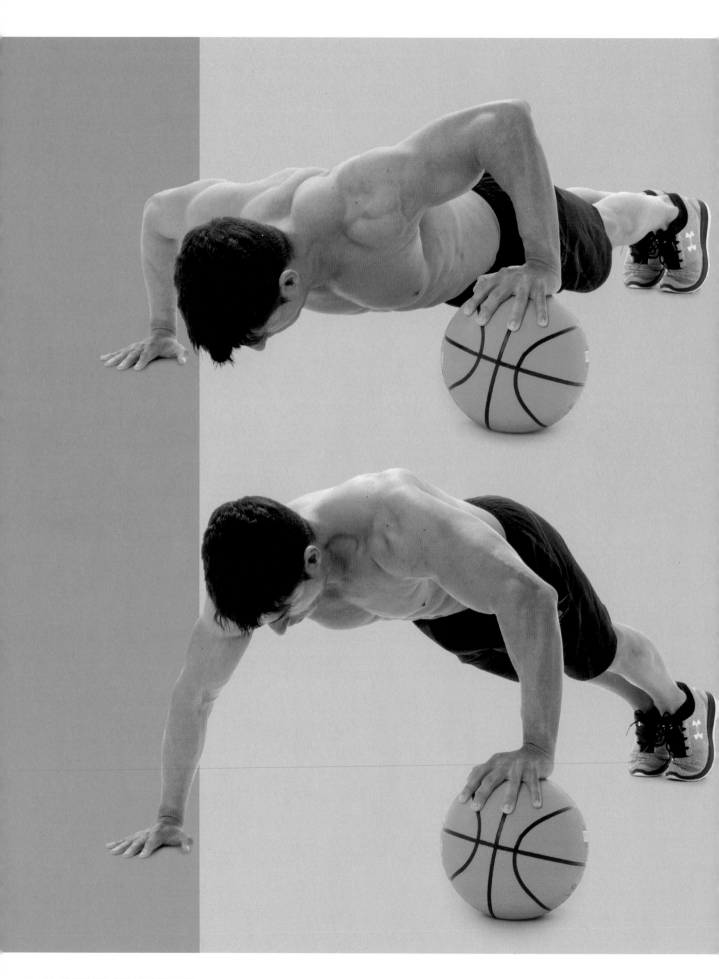

Routines

In this section, we present three training routines at the beginner, intermediate, and advanced levels. These example routines are only guidelines and each athlete should adapt them to his or her abilities and tastes, with careful consideration of any problems that may be present, such as prior injuries, recovery rhythms, etc. The routines that appear on the following pages can be used as a good way to begin, a source of ideas, or just a helpful change for athletes with experience. They are designed to complete a 7-day cycle for which you should take Saturday and Sunday as rest days. One or two rest days per week are desirable; you can choose which days you prefer. Each routine includes principal exercises, where only the number of the exercise is shown, along with its variations, whether these are of lesser, similar or greater difficulty, in which case, the number of the exercise and the symbol for the corresponding variant will appear.

In some exercises, there are a fixed number of repetitions per series (ex.: 4 sets of 12 repetitions); in others, this number is different (ex.: 3 sets of 12-10-8 repetitions respectively). There may also be a range of approximate repetitions (ex.: 3 sets of 8 to 12 repetitions), and occasionally, you may be asked to do the maximum number of repetitions in each series (ex.: 3 sets of maximum repetitions). In this last case, remember that if the number of series you can execute is less than 6 or greater than 20, this means that the difficulty is either too high or too low and you should adjust one of the parameters of the exercise (weight, inclination, etc.). Do not forget to pay attention to the recommendations and training principles that we provide in the early pages of this work, since they will help you to interpret the routines or modify them and design your own routines at any given time.

Beginner

MONDAY

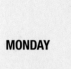

41	PAGE 125	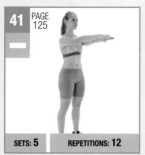
SETS: 5	REPETITIONS: 12	

50	PAGE 143	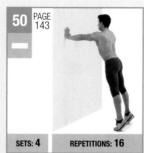
SETS: 4	REPETITIONS: 16	

09	PAGE 61	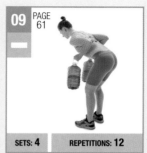
SETS: 4	REPETITIONS: 12	

23	PAGE 89	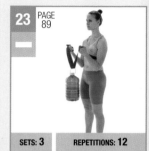
SETS: 3	REPETITIONS: 12	

TUESDAY — REST DAY

WEDNESDAY

42	PAGE 127	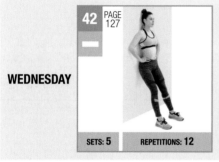
SETS: 5	REPETITIONS: 12	

50	PAGE 142	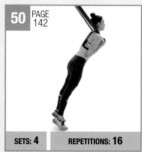
SETS: 4	REPETITIONS: 16	

12	PAGE 67	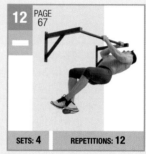
SETS: 4	REPETITIONS: 12	

25	PAGE 93	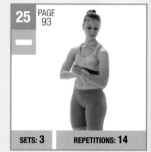
SETS: 3	REPETITIONS: 14	

THURSDAY — REST DAY

FRIDAY

43	PAGE 129	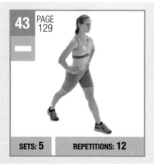
SETS: 5	REPETITIONS: 12	

49	PAGE 141	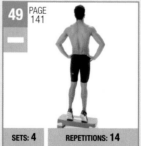
SETS: 4	REPETITIONS: 14	

11	PAGE 64	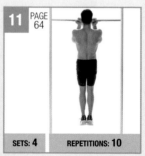
SETS: 4	REPETITIONS: 10	

24	PAGE 90	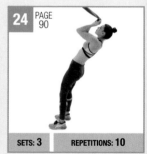
SETS: 3	REPETITIONS: 10	

SATURDAY — REST DAY

SUNDAY — REST DAY

01 PAGE 44 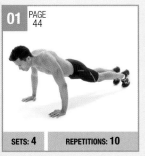 SETS: 4 — REPETITIONS: 10	**17** PAGE 77 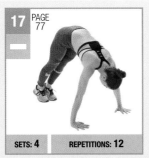 SETS: 4 — REPETITIONS: 12	**26** PAGE 95 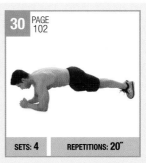 SETS: 3 — REPETITIONS: 12	**30** PAGE 102 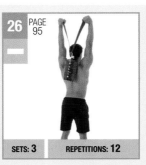 SETS: 4 — REPETITIONS: 20″	**MONDAY**

REST DAY | **TUESDAY**

04 PAGE 51 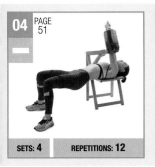 SETS: 4 — REPETITIONS: 12	**18** PAGE 78 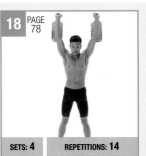 SETS: 4 — REPETITIONS: 14	**27** PAGE 97 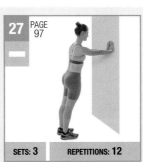 SETS: 3 — REPETITIONS: 12	**31** PAGE 105 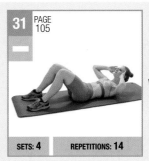 SETS: 4 — REPETITIONS: 14	**WEDNESDAY**

REST DAY | **THURSDAY**

03 PAGE 49 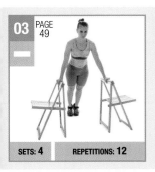 SETS: 4 — REPETITIONS: 12	**21** PAGE 84 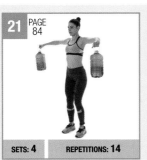 SETS: 4 — REPETITIONS: 14	**28** PAGE 99 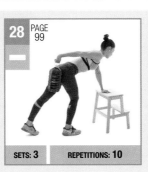 SETS: 3 — REPETITIONS: 10	**32** PAGE 107 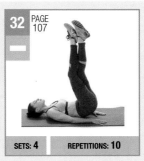 SETS: 4 — REPETITIONS: 10	**FRIDAY**

REST DAY | **SATURDAY**

REST DAY | **SUNDAY**

Intermediate

MONDAY

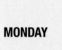 10 | PAGE 63
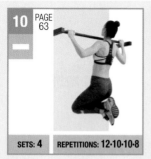
SETS: 4 | REPETITIONS: 12·10·10·8

09 | PAGE 60
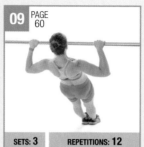
SETS: 3 | REPETITIONS: 12

03 | PAGE 48
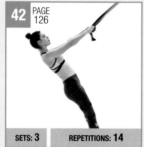
SETS: 4 | REPETITIONS: 10

05 | PAGE 53 ✚
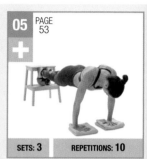
SETS: 3 | REPETITIONS: 10

TUESDAY

41 | PAGE 124
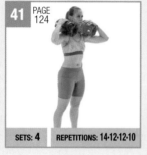
SETS: 4 | REPETITIONS: 14·12·12·10

42 | PAGE 126
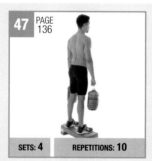
SETS: 3 | REPETITIONS: 14

47 | PAGE 136
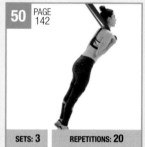
SETS: 4 | REPETITIONS: 10

50 | PAGE 142
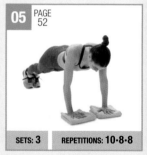
SETS: 3 | REPETITIONS: 20

WEDNESDAY — REST DAY

THURSDAY

11 | PAGE 64
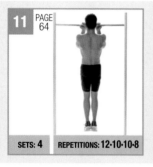
SETS: 4 | REPETITIONS: 12·10·10·8

08 | PAGE 58
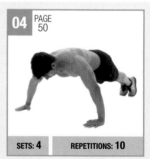
SETS: 4 | REPETITIONS: 12

04 | PAGE 50
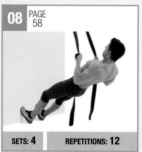
SETS: 4 | REPETITIONS: 10

05 | PAGE 52

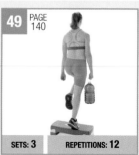
SETS: 3 | REPETITIONS: 10·8·8

FRIDAY

43 | PAGE 128
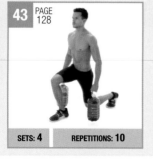
SETS: 4 | REPETITIONS: 10

45 | PAGE 132
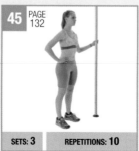
SETS: 3 | REPETITIONS: 10

48 | PAGE 139 ✚
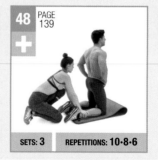
SETS: 3 | REPETITIONS: 10·8·6

49 | PAGE 140
SETS: 3 | REPETITIONS: 12

SATURDAY — REST DAY

SUNDAY — REST DAY

MONDAY

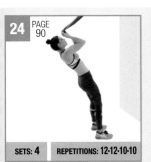
24 PAGE 90
SETS: **4** | REPETITIONS: **12·12·10·10**

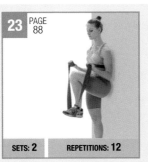
23 PAGE 88
SETS: **2** | REPETITIONS: **12**

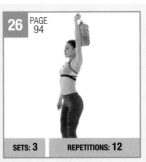
26 PAGE 94
SETS: **3** | REPETITIONS: **12**

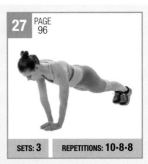
27 PAGE 96
SETS: **3** | REPETITIONS: **10·8·8**

TUESDAY

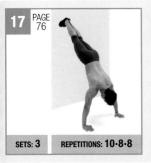
17 PAGE 76
SETS: **3** | REPETITIONS: **10·8·8**

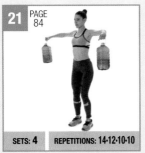
21 PAGE 84
SETS: **4** | REPETITIONS: **14·12·10·10**

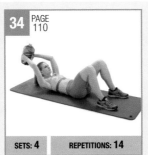
34 PAGE 110
SETS: **4** | REPETITIONS: **14**

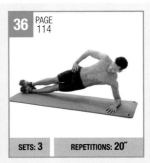
36 PAGE 114
SETS: **3** | REPETITIONS: **20″**

WEDNESDAY

REST DAY

THURSDAY

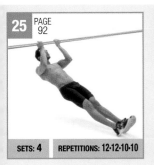
25 PAGE 92
SETS: **4** | REPETITIONS: **12·12·10·10**

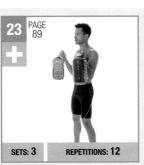

23 PAGE 89
SETS: **3** | REPETITIONS: **12**

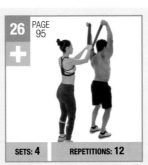

26 PAGE 95
SETS: **4** | REPETITIONS: **12**

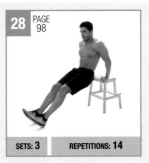
28 PAGE 98
SETS: **3** | REPETITIONS: **14**

FRIDAY

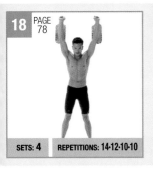
18 PAGE 78
SETS: **4** | REPETITIONS: **14·12·10·10**

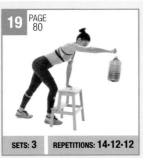
19 PAGE 80
SETS: **3** | REPETITIONS: **14·12·12**

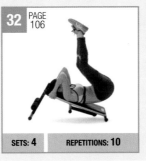
32 PAGE 106
SETS: **4** | REPETITIONS: **10**

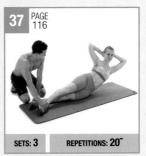
37 PAGE 116
SETS: **3** | REPETITIONS: **20″**

SATURDAY

REST DAY

SUNDAY

REST DAY

Advanced

MONDAY

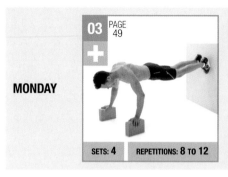

SETS: **4** | REPETITIONS: **8 TO 12**

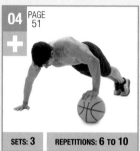

SETS: **3** | REPETITIONS: **6 TO 10**

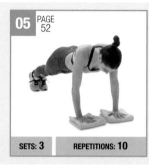

SETS: **3** | REPETITIONS: **10**

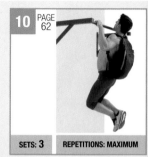

SETS: **3** | REPETITIONS: **MAXIMUM**

TUESDAY

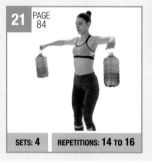

SETS: **4** | REPETITIONS: **14 TO 16**

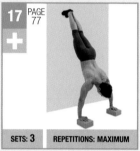

SETS: **3** | REPETITIONS: **MAXIMUM**

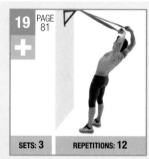

SETS: **3** | REPETITIONS: **12**

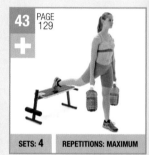

SETS: **4** | REPETITIONS: **MAXIMUM**

WEDNESDAY | REST DAY

THURSDAY

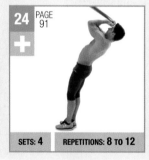

SETS: **4** | REPETITIONS: **8 TO 12**

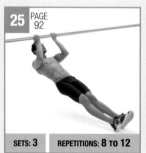

SETS: **3** | REPETITIONS: **8 TO 12**

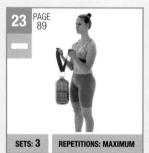

SETS: **3** | REPETITIONS: **MAXIMUM**

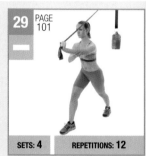

SETS: **4** | REPETITIONS: **12**

FRIDAY

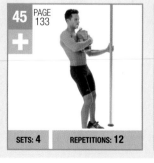

SETS: **4** | REPETITIONS: **12**

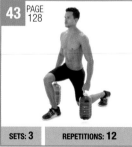

SETS: **3** | REPETITIONS: **12**

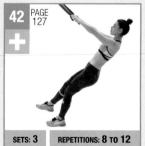

SETS: **3** | REPETITIONS: **8 TO 12**

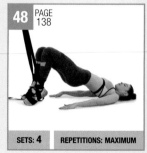

SETS: **4** | REPETITIONS: **MAXIMUM**

SATURDAY | REST DAY

SUNDAY | REST DAY

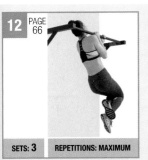 **12** PAGE 66 — SETS: 3 — REPETITIONS: MAXIMUM	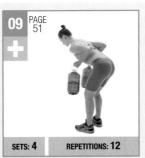 **09** ✚ PAGE 51 — SETS: 4 — REPETITIONS: 12	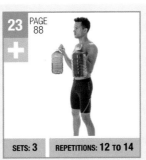 **23** ✚ PAGE 88 — SETS: 3 — REPETITIONS: 12 TO 14	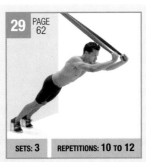 **29** PAGE 62 — SETS: 3 — REPETITIONS: 10 TO 12	**MONDAY**

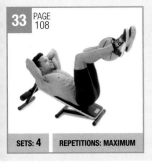 **33** PAGE 108 — SETS: 4 — REPETITIONS: MAXIMUM	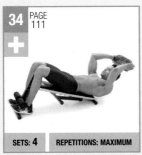 **34** ✚ PAGE 111 — SETS: 4 — REPETITIONS: MAXIMUM	**TUESDAY**

REST DAY	**WEDNESDAY**

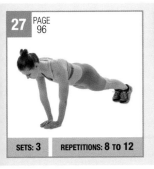 **27** PAGE 96 — SETS: 3 — REPETITIONS: 8 TO 12	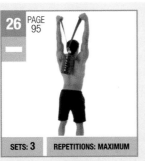 **26** PAGE 95 — SETS: 3 — REPETITIONS: MAXIMUM	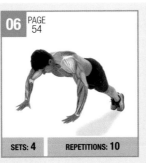 **06** PAGE 54 — SETS: 4 — REPETITIONS: 10	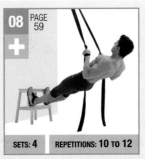 **08** ✚ PAGE 59 — SETS: 4 — REPETITIONS: 10 TO 12	**THURSDAY**

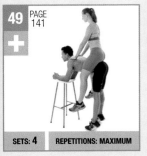 **49** ✚ PAGE 141 — SETS: 4 — REPETITIONS: MAXIMUM	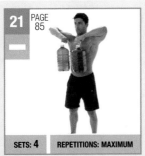 **21** — PAGE 85 — SETS: 4 — REPETITIONS: MAXIMUM	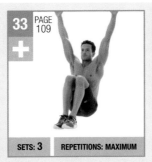 **33** ✚ PAGE 109 — SETS: 3 — REPETITIONS: MAXIMUM	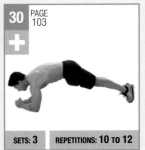 **30** ✚ PAGE 103 — SETS: 3 — REPETITIONS: 10 TO 12	**FRIDAY**

REST DAY	**SATURDAY**

REST DAY	**SUNDAY**

Bibliography

Ahtiainen, Juha P. et al. "Short vs Long rest period between the sets in hypertrophic resistance training: Influence on muscle strength, size and hormonal adaptations in trained men." *Journal of Strength and Conditioning Research* (2005), 19(3), 572-582.

Amirthaligam, Theban et al. "Effects of a modified german volume training program on muscular hypertrophy and strength." *Journal of Strength and Conditioning Research* (2017),DOI: 10.1519/ JSC.0000000000001747.

Buresh, Robet; Berg, Kris y French, Jeffren. "The effect of resistive exercise rest interval on hormonal response, strength and hypertrophy with training." *Journal of Strength and Conditioning Research* (2009), 23: 62-71.

Campos, Gerson E. R. et al. "Muscular adaptations in response to three different resistance-training regimens: specificity of repetition maximum training zones." *European Journal of Applied Physiology*, DOI 10.1007/s00421-002-0681-6.

Cribb, Paul J. y Hayes, Alan. *Effects of supplement timing and resistance exercise on skeletal muscle hypertrophy.* American College of Sports Medicine, 2006.

Esmarck, B. et al. "Timing of postexercise protein intake is important for muscle hypertrophy with resistance training in elderly humans." *Journal of Physiology* (2001), 535.1: 301-311.

Flann, Kyle L. "Muscle damage and muscle remodeling: no pain, no gain?" *Journal of Experimental Biology* (2011), 214, 674-679.

Folland, Jonathan P. y Williams, Alun G. "The adaptations to strength training. Morphological and neurological contributions to increased strength." *Sports Medicine* (2007), 37 (2): 145-168.

Fry, Andrew C. "The role of resistance exercise intensity on muscle fibre adaptations." *Sports Medicine* (2004), 10: 663-679.

García Ramos, Amador et al. "Mechanical and metabolic responses to traditional and cluster set configurations in the bench press exercises." *Journal of Strength and Conditioning Research* (2017), DOI: 10.1519/ JSC.0000000000002302.

Hayes, Alana y Cribb, Paul J. *Effect of whey protein isolate on strength, body composition and muscle hypertrophy during resistance training.* School of Biomedical Sciences, Victoria University, 2008.

Hickson, Robert C. "Simultaneously training for strength and endurance". *European Journal of Applied Physiology* (1980), 45: 255-263.

Helms, Eric. *Effects of training-induced hormonal changes on muscular hypertrophy.* An Annotated Bibliography by Eric Helms, 2010.

Hwang, Paul y Willoughby, Darryn S. "Mechanisms behind blood flow restricted training and its effect towards muscle growth." *Journal of Strength and Conditioning Research* (2017), DOI: 10.1519/ JSC.0000000000002384.

Kalyn, Ashley. *Manual de ejercicio con el peso corporal.* Paidotribo, Barcelona, 2016.

Kraemer, William J. et al. *Adaptaciones musculares como respuesta a tres regimens de entrenamiento de fuerza. Especificidad de las zonas de entrenamiento de repeticiones máximas.* PubliCE, 2002.

Krieger, James W. "Single vs. Multiple sets of resistance exercise for muscle hypertrophy: a meta-analysis." *Journal of Strength and Conditioning Research* (2010), 24(4): 1,150-1,159.

Loenneke, Jeremy P. "Skeletal muscle hypertrophy: How important is exercise intensity?" *Journal of Trainology* (2012), 2:28-3.

Lundberg, Tommy. *The effects of aerobic exercise on human skeletal muscle adaptations to resistance exercise.* Thesis for Doctoral degree. Östersund, Mid Sweeden University, 2014.

Merí, Àlex. *Fundamentos de la fisiología de la actividad física y el deporte.* Médica panamericana, 2005.

Miller, Ryan M. et al. "Effects of blood flow restriction combined with post activation potentiation stimuli on jump performance in recreationally active males." *Journal of Strength and Conditioning Research* (2017), DOI: 10.1519/ JSC.0000000000002110.

Mitchell, Cameron J. *Muscular and systemic correlates of resistance training-induced muscle hypertrophy.* Plos One (2013), vol. 8, n.º 10.

Moraes, Evelin. "Relationship between repetitions and selected percentage of one repetition maximum in trained and untrained adolescent subjects." *Journal of Exercise Physiology* (2014), vol. 17, n.º 2.

Ogasawa, Riki et al. "Low-Load Bench Press Training to Fatigue Results in Muscle Hypertrophy Similar to High-Load Bench Press Training." *International Journal of Clinical Medicine* (2013), 4, 114-121.

Ogborn, Dan y Schoenfeld, Brad J. "The role of fiber types in muscle hypertrophy: implications for loading strategies." *Journal of Strength and Conditioning Research* (2014), 36 (2): 20-25.

Rahmidi, Rahman et al. "The effect of different rest intervals between sets on the training volume of male athletes." *Physical Education and Sport* (2007), 5: 37-46.

Schoenfeld, Brad. *Science and development of muscle hypertrophy.* Human Kinetics, 2016.

Schoenfeld, Brad y Grgic, Jozo. "Can drop sets training enhance muscle growth?" *Journal of Strength and Conditioning Research* (2017), DOI: 10.1519/ SSC.0000000000000366.

Schoenfeld, Brad J. "Potential mechanisms for a role of metabolic stress in hypertrophic adaptations to resistance training." *Sports Medicine* (2013), DOI 10.1007/ s40279-013-0017-1.

Schoenfeld, Brad J. "The mechanisms of muscle hypertrophy and their application to resistance training." *Global Fitness Services* (2010), vol. 24, n.º 10.

Schoenfeld, Brad J. "The use of specialized training techniques to maximize muscle hypertrophy." *Journal of Strength and Conditioning Research* (2011), 33 (4): 60-65.

Senna, Gilmar et al. "Influence of two different rest interval lengths in resistance training sessions for upper and lower body." *Journal of Sports and Medicine* (2008), 8: 197-202.

Short, Kevin R. et al. "Age and aerobic exercise training effects on whole body and muscle protein metabolism." *American Journal of Physiology-Endocrinology and Metabolism* (2003), 286: 92-101.

Tiago Fernandes, Úrsula. "Sygnaling pathways that mediate skeletal muscle hypertrophy: Effects of exercise training." *FPESP* (2010), 50048-1 y n.º. 2009/18370-3.

Tomohiro, Yasuda. "Effects of low-intensity bench press training with restricted arm muscle blood flow on chest muscle hypertrophy: a pilot study." *Clinical Physiology and Functional Imaging* (2010), 30: 338-343.